CHEERLEADING CONDITIONING FOR PEAK PERFORMANCE

Elaine Hart
Chris Kirby
The International Cheerleading Foundation, Inc.

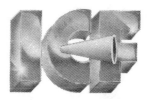

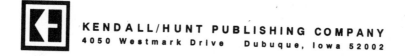
KENDALL/HUNT PUBLISHING COMPANY
4050 Westmark Drive   Dubuque, Iowa 52002

TABLE OF CONTENTS

INTRODUCTION

TO OUR READERS . . .

Attaining excellence is a life long pursuit for all achievers. In cheerleading, excellence is seen when a squad develops an enthusiastic, positive atmosphere of spirit and pride within and around a school. Cheerleaders achieve this goal through performances and crowd leadership at various games and school events such as pep rallies. Successful crowd leadership is a tricky task involving turning around negative cheering, rousing an inactive crowd, and unifying and leading a cheering audience to best impact the team. Cheers, tumbling, jumps, and other cheering skills are all used to develop crowd leadership. Attaining excellence or "peak performance" in each of these skills will lead to excellence in cheerleading.

Proper **technique** and **conditioning** are both necessary for peak performance of your cheerleading skills. **Technique training,** which teaches you how to execute a skill, has always been the focus of cheerleading instructors, manuals, workshops, etc. **Conditioning training,** however, has been almost non-existent and therefore is the motivation behind this book. Although you will find a great deal of information in the following chapters, you may not be ready for all the details! In order to learn what you need and you don't get "bogged down", let's examine what's in the book, who the readers are, and how best to use the information.

WHO'S READING THIS BOOK?

Across America over 600,000 cheerleaders and nearly 50,000 coaches are involved in cheerleading activities. These numbers do not include the thousands of cheerleaders in other parts of the world such as Japan, Canada and England! Due to the fact that so many people participate in cheerleading and because conditioning is a vital part of athletic excellence, it is easy to see why a book on conditioning is well over due!

All kinds of people are interested in improving cheerleading skills including junior high, senior high and collegiate cheerleaders; beginner to advanced cheerleaders; first time and experienced coaches; plus, athletic trainers and medical personnel who are interested in helping cheerleaders improve their athletic performance. Many male and female collegiate (or collegiate bound) cheerleaders will use the text as a guide in developing a high powered, athletic workout. These people may be seeking scholarships in cheerleading and they are determined to advance their skills to the highest level possible. At the other end of the spectrum we find many beginning cheerleaders and coaches trying to establish a basic conditioning program that will give their squad a solid foundation for improving skills and overall performance in a safe and simple manner.

Each of our readers' needs are different; however, everyone involve in cheerleading is interested in safe, effective performance and that's what conditioning is all about. The key idea here is **read what you need** . . . and don't "overload" by trying to read the entire book all at one time!

CHAPTER TOPICS

Chapter 1 and 2, "UNDERSTANDING FITNESS" and "DEVELOPING YOUR WORK-OUT." The first two chapters will give you and your squad a **basic understanding of fitness** as it relates to cheerleading — why it is important, what fitness means and how to initiate your program. In chapter 1 you'll gain a basic understanding of the different areas or "components of fitness" and how they relate to cheerleading skill development and performance. The chapter begins by examining the need for fitness: strength, power, endurance, nutrition, body composition and mental skills. Chapter 2 focuses on **how to develop a workout.** Key principles for productive workouts are discussed along with goal setting, medical exams, motivation and sample workout schedules.

Chapters 3-7, "ENDURANCE," "STRENGTH AND POWER," "FLEXIBILITY," "NUTRITION AND BODY COMPOSITION," and "PYSCHOLOGICAL SKILLS."

Each of the above listed chapters focuses on one specific area or "component" of fitness and how it affects your cheering skills. Beginning cheerleaders should not try to "take" in all this information at once nor should those of you who are not ready to learn the in-depth, inner-workings of the body. Regardless of your level, make sure to read the key concepts outlined in these chapters so you will understand how each fitness component affects you cheerleading skills. Step-by-step exercise photographs and instructions are included in chapters 3-5.

Chapters 8-11, "JUMPS," "GYMNASTICS," "PARTNER STUNTS," and "DANCE."

Have you ever wondered why — after learning and practicing proper technique — your skills still don't look as good as you want them? Up to now, all you have been taught is to practice until perfect, right? Wrong! It is not that simple.

What about conditioning for a specific skill? How does your level of endurance, strength, power, and flexibility relate to the jump or the stunt you are trying to master? Chapters 8-11 study each skill area and focus on **conditioning for specific skills**. Here again we recommend you **don't overload** by trying to read everything at once; instead, you may want to skim these four chapters to understand the basic concepts. You can then refer back to a chapter when you are ready to work on a specific skill.

Chapters 12 and 13, "EVALUATING YOUR PROGRESS," and "INJURY PREVENTION."

We finish our book with specific testing procedures to determine how successful your workout is and some important tips on safety and injury prevention for cheerleaders. The **evaluation chapter** contains both simple means of measuring your progress (your captain or coach can do these) as well as in depth, exact systems that a physical therapist or sports training may need to administer. And, as you can imagine, injury prevention techniques should be read and understood by coaches and cheerleaders alike in hopes of keeping cheerleading in a positive, safe, and rewarding activity.

Conditioning is a key factor in peak performance as well as injury prevention. **Cheerleading Conditioning for Peak Performance** is the first book of its kind and is the result of many hours of research and training. We are excited to offer you the information and step-by-step conditioning programs that will enable you to pursue athletic excellence as a cheerleader!

Elaine Hart and Chris Kirby

IMPORTANT INDIVIDUAL MUSCLES

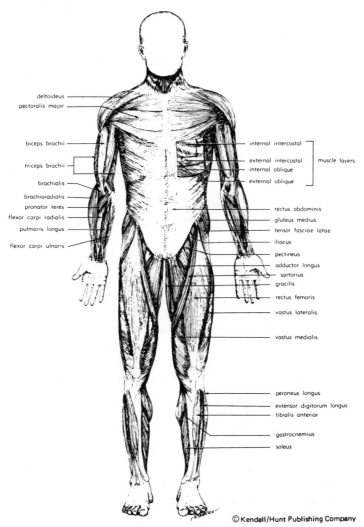

Figure 0-1. Important Individual Muscles.

ARMS

Triceps. The triceps, which are located in the back of the upper arm, help you lift above your head, push, and extend or straighten your arms. Strength Exercises: pushing and straightening movement or your upper arm.

Biceps. These muscles are in the front of your upper arms. Their work is opposite from the triceps. They bend your elbow to help you pull and lift. Strength Exercises: twisting and bending.

Forearms Muscles. This group of muscles between your wrist and elbow controls all wrist movement and helps you in gripping. Strength Exercises: grip arm bending.

SHOULDERS

Deltoids. Deltoids are your shoulder muscles. The front, middle, and rear deltoids assist in moving your arms either forward or backward and in lifting them to the side. Strength Exercises: arm raising and overhead movement.

ABDOMINALS

Rectus Abdominals. The muscular area on the front and sides of your trunk (between the sternum and pelvis) are your abdominals. Strength Exercises: sit-ups, leg raises, knee-in movements.

External Oblique Abdominals. Located on the lower sides of your waist, these muscles assist with waist twisting and bending.

CHEST

Pectorals. The pectoral muscles (chest muscles) pull your arms across your body laterally and help when you push your arms to the front. Strength Exercises: drawing arms across your body and horizontal pressing.

BACK

Trapezius. Located in the upper back and on each side of the neck, these large triangular muscles cover most of the area of your upper back. The trapezius lift your shoulders and assist the deltoids and arm muscles in various movements of the arms and shoulders. Strength Exercises: upward pulling and shoulder shrugging movement.

Latissimus dorsi. Wide, fan-like back muscles that laterally cover most of the back. The "lats" work with your arm muscles in most pulling movements. Strength Exercises: rowing and pulling movements.

Lower back muscles. (Including spinal erector muscles) Helps raise the upper body from a bent over position. This is an area of weakness for many cheerleaders. The lower-back muscles are essential for good posture, alignment and balance.

LEGS AND BUTTOCKS

Adductors and Abductors. The inside (adductors) and the outside (abductors) of your thighs.

Gluteus maximus. The muscular area covering your seat. The buttocks muscles are powerful in bringing about a backward movement of the thighs. Strength Exercises: lunging, stooping, leg raising.

Quadriceps. Your "quads" are the large muscle groups that make up most of the front of your thighs. Quadricep muscles straighten the knee.

Biceps femoris. Commonly called "hamstrings," leg biceps are located on the back of the thigh. Working just opposite from the quadriceps, the leg biceps bend your knee. Strength Exercises: bending forward and stretching, raising lower leg to buttocks.

Gastrocnemius. The calf muscles, located on the backs of your lower legs, between the knee and ankle, lift your heel off the ground and initiate the walking movement. Strength Exercises: raising and lowering on toes.

UNDERSTANDING FITNESS
Chapter One

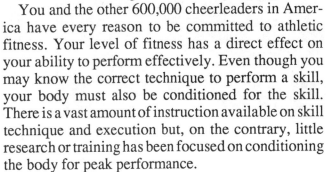

LOOKING FIT OR BEING FIT?

Fitness information is everywhere — books, television, magazines — it's a popular subject! The general public has recently learned of the health benefits associated with keeping fit and athletes have long been aware that their fitness level has a direct effect on their performance. But, what about cheerleaders? What about fitness as it relates to a cheerleader's performance?

As a crowd leader, performer, and school representative, you are in the public eye and are concerned with "looking fit." The question is, are we only interested in "looking fit" or actually "being fit"?

You and the other 600,000 cheerleaders in America have every reason to be committed to athletic fitness. Your level of fitness has a direct effect on your ability to perform effectively. Even though you may know the correct technique to perform a skill, your body must also be conditioned for the skill. There is a vast amount of instruction available on skill technique and execution but, on the contrary, little research or training has been focused on conditioning the body for peak performance.

The image of a cheerleader has not always been complimentary — you know the cliches: "In it for the popularity, unsure or unconcerned with which team has the ball, short skirts, lots of simple jumps and silly movement that require no real athletic skill" . . . and the list goes on! Cheerleaders have always been interested in looking the part; however, only in recent years as cheerleaders began taking pride in their physical ability has an interest developed in serious conditioning for athletic performance.

WHY CONDITION?

Your squad's athletic fitness is a key ingredient in developing crowd rapport and respect. Proper conditioning allows you to perform at your athletic peak from the start to finish of each game you cheer. Following your conditioning efforts, don't be surprised when you notice the new sense of athletic pride developing within each member of your squad.

No one wants to return to the days of old and frankly, the crowds would never respond to that, would they? For those of you who are committed to developing your cheering skills to your full potential in the safest, most efficient way possible, this book is for you! Cheerleaders everywhere are taking their role as spirit leaders seriously and, by understanding and practicing the conditioning guidelines in this book, you'll be on your way to peak cheerleading performance.

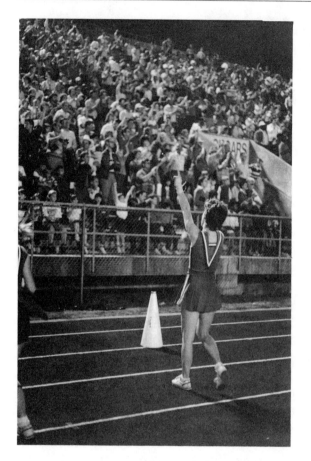

DEFINITION OF FITNESS

Fitness can be described as the capacity to carry out everyday activities without excessive fatigue and with enough energy left over to deal with any potential emergencies that might arise. Our high-tech world doesn't demand much fitness; especially not enough to perform physically demanding cheering skills. As athletes, cheerleaders should view fitness as the optimization of health, instead of the "minimum daily requirement" necessary to fit into that uniform! This means that health is not only the absence of disease, but a dynamic state in which you are able to take your body to its highest physical potential.

FOUR BASIC COMPONENTS OF FITNESS

The four key areas of "components" or a cheerleader's physical fitness are: 1) endurance (both cardiorespiratory and muscular), 2) strength and power, 3) flexibility, and 4) nutrition and body composition. Psychological skills are also included in our definition of fitness. Each of these fitness components plays a vital role in your overall fitness level and in the physical and mental requirements of cheerleading performance. Let's take a quick look at each component of fitness as it relates to cheerleading.

"Our squad is in good condition. We're aerobically fit and we're all pretty strong but we still have trouble getting our kicks up as high as we want. How do we pin point what's wrong?"

ENDURANCE

The capacity of a muscle or group of muscles to exert force repeatedly over time refers to its muscular endurance. Likewise, cardiorespiratory endurance refers to the ability of the heart, blood vessels and lungs to deliver nutrients and oxygen, and to remove metabolic waste for extended periods. Muscular endurance can contribute to your ability to perform high level tumbling or to hold a solid position in a pyramid or partner stunt. A highly conditioned cardiorespiratory system is helpful for executing skills near the end of a game, when performing long routines that incorporate many skills in succession, and for general energetic performance over an extended period of time.

> *"I know the proper form, but I never seem to have enough time in the air to execute my jump. What type of conditioning exercises can help?"*

STRENGTH AND POWER

Strength is the capacity of muscle(s) to exert the greatest possible force against a resistance. Many times your muscular strength is a major part of cheerleading; however, cheerleading is primarily a power oriented activity. Power is the force created over a distance per unit of time. It also is the ability to project an object or body rapidly through space. Strength will help you create power. The speed of your movement also helps generate muscular power. Imagine performing a perfect toe touch jump or a series of back handsprings ending in a beautiful back layout! The generation of muscular power would enable you to perform these exciting skills.

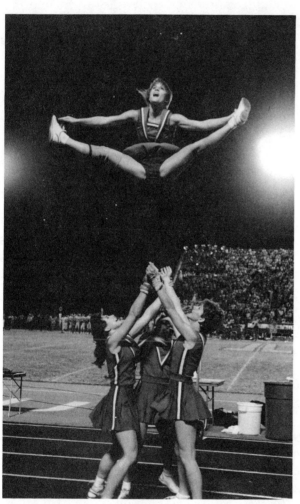

> *"Our squad is in good condition. We're aerobically fit and we're all pretty strong but we still have trouble getting our kicks up as high as we want. How do we pin point what's wrong?"*

FLEXIBILITY

Most cheering skills require good flexibility. Think about it. Splits, kicks, most jumps and gymnastics, heel stretches in your stunts and many dance moves involve flexibility. The "range of motion" or degree of movement about a particular joint describes its flexibility. The range of movement possible involves many factors; the amount of muscular and fat (adipose) tissue surrounding the joint, the angle at which muscles insert (via tendons) into the bone, the laxity of ligaments and the bone to bone interactions.

Flexibility can be divided into two types: **static and dynamic**. Your ability to reach the split position is determined by the static flexibility of your hip flexors and extensors. In contrast, the type of flexibility used more frequently is dynamic flexibility, which is the resistance to motion displayed by a particular joint. An example of dynamic flexibility is a pike jump or an aerial walkover.

"My squad has horrendous eating habits. They either 'crash diet' or consume lots of junk food. Can eating habits affect our squad's performance level?"

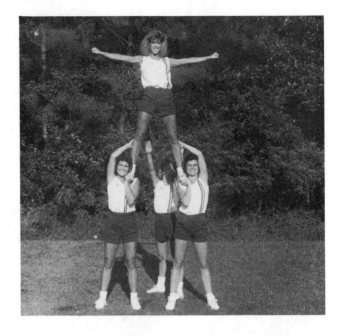

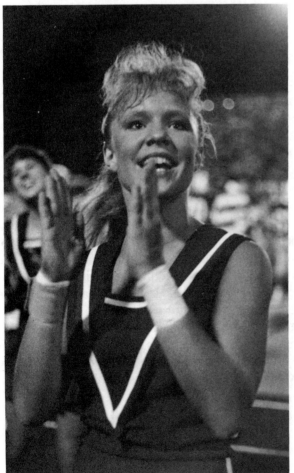

NUTRITION

Nutrition is often thought of as the **"science of foods."** This field deals not only with the composition of foods (e.g., the amount of fat or specific vitamins found in a particular food), but also the way the body uses foods to create energy for work, repair tissues, produce substances which control physiological function and many other uses critical to maintaining life.

Your nutritional health plays a major role in your overall fitness and in your cheerleading performance. You and your squad need good nutritional habits in order to gain the greatest possible benefits from physical conditioning, to enhance your recovery from exercise and to cheer at your peak throughout the entire year. Be sure to read about common eating disorders that can cause even worse problems than poor eating habits!

> *"Every year I have problems determining weight guidelines for my squad. What is safe? What is effective? What is fair? Aren't weight charts out of date?"*

BODY COMPOSITION

Body composition is the relative amount of fat and lean tissue that make up your total body weight. Instead of relaying on scale weight, it is more important to look at the composition of your weight. This vital component of fitness affects every area of your performance and only by determining your body composition can you find out the amount of functional tissue versus "excess baggage" that you can use to perform your cheerleading skills.

> *"It's hard for me to learn back walkovers and back handsprings. I am afraid of going backwards and I don't know how to control my fear."*

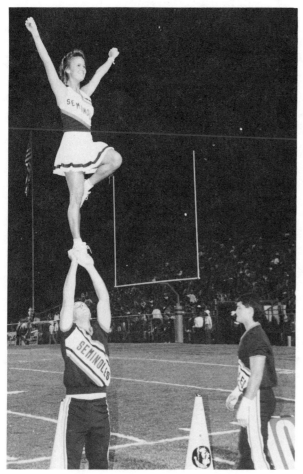

PSYCHOLOGICAL SKILLS

Many athletes and coaches do not realize the impact mental conditioning plays in skill development. According to an expert in the field, Dr. Jean Williams, the goal of psychological training in athletics is "learning to consistently create the ideal climate that unleashes those physical skills which allow athletes to perform at their best." It has been said of many athletic activities that success is 90 percent mental and 10 percent physical and cheerleading is no exception. Basic training in visualization, concentration, etc. will make a big difference in the way you and your squad cheer together!

There are many benefits from being physically and mentally fit for cheerleading including reducing the potential for injuries. Hopefully, your interest in fitness and your initiation of a squad fitness program will result in a lifetime commitment to dynamic health. After all, when you think about the athletic activity cheerleading has become, it doesn't really make sense for cheerleaders to be anything but fit, now does it?

DEVELOPING YOUR WORKOUT
Chapter Two

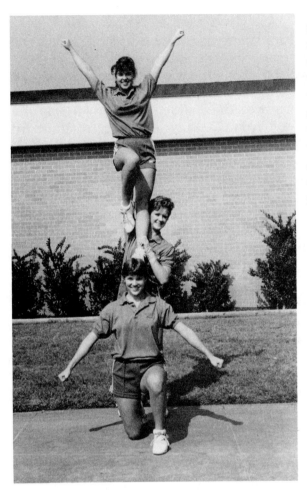

Have you ever begun a project that initially seemed like a good idea but ended up being a big mistake? You know the feeling, don't you? What once was a good idea somehow evolves into a frustrating, unproductive undertaking. Although you will never make progress if you don't begin, it is common to see people plunge into an activity without proper planning. Our goal is to help you **get fitness results** without wasting precious time and energy. Once you understand the principles of conditioning outlined in this book, you will be ready to develop a specific workout. Be sure to familiarize yourself with each of the workout planning factors outlined in this chapter. They are of vital importance to help you get results.

WORKOUT PLANNING FACTORS

Several factors need to be considered as you put together the best workout for your squad. These factors include:
1) Goals.
2) Current fitness level and needs.
3) Practice time and facilities.
4) Motivation.
5) Periodization.

GOAL SETTING

> *"Everyone on our squad has decided to make a commitment to get in shape, but we don't know how to get started. We know we don't want to be wasting our time with a program that doesn't accomplish much!"*

Goal setting requires knowing what you hope to accomplish, by when, and how. To set your fitness goals, you first need to **educate** yourself about fitness, then **evaluate** your current level of fitness and performance abilities, and finally **determine where you want to be** after a given period of time. Set up your long term goals (six months, one year, two years, etc.) by considering both your personal goals and aspirations as well as your squad's goals.

Once you know your long term fitness and performance objectives, set up a series of short term, attainable goals. These short term goals will be your "plan of attack" or the actual steps you will follow to achieve your goals. Be sure to put your goals in writing and, once your workout is underway, remember to evaluate your progress periodically so you can make any necessary adjustments to your program.

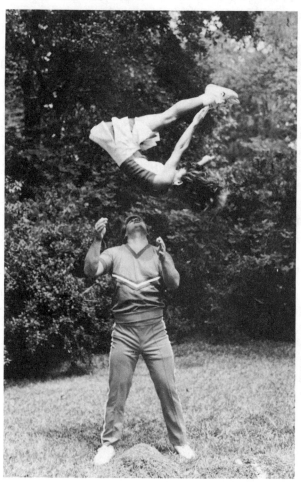

CURRENT FITNESS LEVEL

How fit are you? To develop a safe conditioning program, first determine your current fitness level. Include a complete **medical examination** to find out the general status of your health. An examination by a **certified athletic trainer** will help determine if you have any limitations resulting from orthopedic, muscular or neurologic deficiencies. These examinations ideally should be followed by an evaluation of your fitness level based on cheerleading standards. This type of fitness evaluation (discussed in chapter 12) will help you determine your needs in strength and power, endurance, and flexibility.

PRACTICE TIME AND FACILITIES

The time you devote to conditioning will have a direct effect on the success of your workout. Since the time available for cheerleading practice is already limited, plan carefully. Keep in mind that **inconsistent workout times often lead to nonexistent workouts,** so plan a realistic program.

How much time should be devoted to actual fitness training versus practicing jumps, gymnastics, stunts, and dance? How do you incorporate conditioning exercises into your normal practice schedule? How much of conditioning should be done as a team versus working out on your own? Your normal practice schedule usually includes working on specific skills (jumps, tumbling, stunts, dance, etc.) along with cheers, chants and complete routine performances. You'll be amazed to find out that once you learn proper technique, **conditioning for a skill cuts down the time it takes to master a skill!** For example, mastering a toe touch jump will be much quicker once you are conditioned to perform a toe touch!

The amount of time available for training will help you determine a **workout schedule** to which you and your squad can commit. You will also need to keep in mind what facilities and equipment are available for your workout (i.e., jump ropes, swimming pool, weights, mats, etc.). Many squads choose to incorporate fitness workouts into each of their normal practices; others alternate conditioning at one practice and practicing skills at the next. Good results are often achieved by incorporating workouts for a given area of fitness at the beginning or end of your regular practice. Also, scheduling days which are devoted solely to conditioning can be a great way of breaking up the monotony of practices late in the season!

We do not recommend that workouts of any type (flexibility, endurance, strength and power, etc.) exceed one to one and one-half hours in duration. It is difficult to maintain adequate physical and mental intensity with overly long workouts (see the Overload Principle, later in this chapter). Also, most squads will find it difficult to devote any more than this amount of time consistently.

MOTIVATION

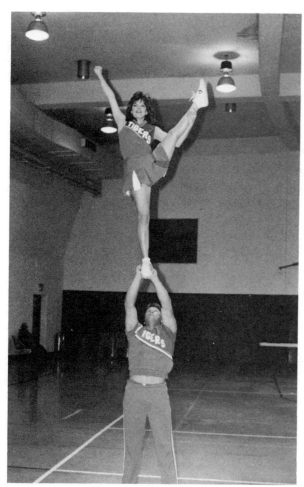

ATTITUDE

Your attitude influences the quality of your workout. The mind set with which we **choose** to enter our workouts is the single greatest determinant of the success or failure of our conditioning program. Cheerleaders who go into a workout expecting results generally achieve them, while those who approach their workouts as an unpleasant fact of life rarely obtain maximal benefit for their efforts.

In order to approach your daily workouts with a desire to give 110 percent physically and mentally, you need to develop a **positive mental attitude (PMA)**. PMA is not just a catchy buzzword, but an overall view of the circumstances and challenges which make up our daily lives enabling us to benefit the most from a given situation.

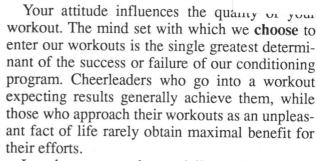

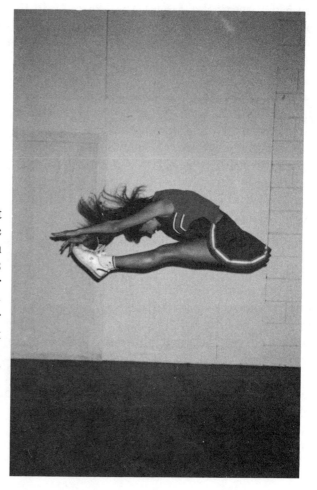

WORKOUT PARTNERS

Although our goal is to approach every workout as another opportunity for progress, some days we allow life's little circumstances to distract us from our purpose in training. It is at these times that it is helpful to have a training partner(s) to bolster our lack of desire and help us achieve a quality workout. Whether you condition with just one partner or your entire squad, we encourage you to work out with someone. **A workout partner is helpful in challenging and encouraging you to give your best during a workout.** Partners are used frequently in many flexibility exercises as well as strength and power training.

ACHIEVEMENT STANDARDS

A great way to provide incentive for improving our physical condition is to set up standards of achievement. Evaluate progress consistently and plan special awards for achievement such as having names placed on the "Cheerleading Conditioning Wall of Fame," giving t-shirts or warm-ups, or recognition in a school. Even though the benefits of improved skill performance and improved overall well-being are great motivators, a little extra positive reinforcement can go a long way!

SELECTING YOUR EXERCISES

The information you obtain from a medical examination and fitness evaluation should be used in conjunction with your goals to determine the **frequency, intensity and duration** of your workouts. Detailed sample exercises are outlined throughout this book and, based on your current fitness level, you will select the exercises that will best help you reach your goals. The sample conditioning workouts at the end of this chapter will give you an idea how to set up your daily program.

WORKOUT VARIATIONS

It is unrealistic to expect to remain in top form year round and improve every day. Using definate exercises for **the same muscle group** is a great way to incorporate variety in your workout. Since the major muscle groups used in cheerleading are the same throughout the conditioning program, be creative in selecting the specific exercises used to train that particular group. The exercises in this book are not the only appropriate exercises available; they may be modified and supplemented for variety and greater specificity to your particular needs.

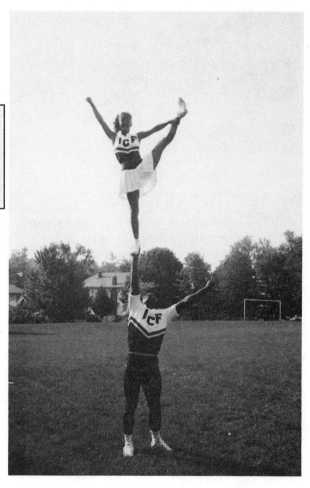

> *"The football coach at our school helped us get started on the conditioning program he uses for his team, but for some reason we didn't notice improvement in our cheerleading skills, even though we seemed to be in better shape."*

SPECIFICITY

Your fitness level will improve primarily in the physiological systems you stress through your exercises. This concept, called specificity, means you must know which skills you are trying to improve and then you must design your workout to improve the areas of fitness associated with that skill. **Exercise(s) must mimic the skill you are trying to develop.** Specificity is the guiding concept throughout this book with the purpose of teaching you how to condition, both generally and for the specific skills you are trying to develop.

PERIODIZATION

> *"Our squad basically cheers year-round. How can we make sure we are at our peak every time we cheer?"*

A cheerleader's season is longer than most sports and involves spring tryouts, summer practice, and fall and winter cheering. How do you remain motivated and at your physical peak throughout the year? A **cycling of training methods and intensities,** called "periodization," is needed to make sure you have the physical capability to achieve peak performance when you need it most. Periodization involves three principles: overload, recovery and reversibility.

OVERLOAD PRINCIPLE

> *"Every year I start practices with some basic conditioning exercises to prepare my squad for camp. But, after a few weeks their improvement seems to stop, even though we are still working just as hard."*

Fitness gains will only be achieved when the physiological systems you are conditioning (e.g., cardiorespiratory, muscular, etc.) are loaded beyond their normal requirements. This is called the "overload principle." For instance, if you want to increase the amount of muscular power (force produced over a distance per unit of time) in your jumps, you must require your muscles to generate either more force at the same speed or the same force at a greater speed than what they normally produce. In addition, the principle of progressive resistance requires that stress must be gradually increased in a particular area of fitness to make sure the system is continually overloaded.

EXERCISE RECOVERY

> *"It seems like every year when we begin to prepare for an important performance, injuries start occurring. Just when we want to be our best, everyone seems exhausted."*

Adequate rest is vital to insure full **recovery** following exercise. You will be wasting time if you attempt to do too much exercise without giving your body time to recover between workouts! Although recovery time varies for each cheerleader and over a wide range of fitness levels, it is essential to your conditioning program. In fact, if you go beyond these limits a state of **overtraining** will occur in which fitness gains for the same amount of exercise actually **decrease** and your potential for injury significantly **increase.** Be sure to read over the suggestions for recognizing the occurrence of overtraining in the evaluation chapter of this book.

PRINCIPLE OF REVERSIBILITY

If you stop training, you will quickly learn about the "principle of reversibility" which is the opposite of overtraining. Since physiological changes happen quickly (several hours to days) cheerleaders need to be consistent in their workouts in order to remain in excellent condition. If you want to maintain your new peak condition, don't quit your workout!

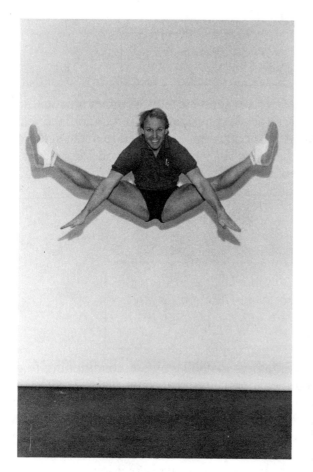

SAMPLE CONDITIONING PROGRAMS

The following workouts are a sample showing you how to apply conditioning principles. Remember, however, that these are generic programs and that it is critical to the success of your individual fitness program to follow the steps outlined previously in this chapter. You will need to refer to chapters (3-6) for details on each component of fitness.

PRE-SEASON

This period lasts approximately five months (April to August) and is characterized by high value and high intensity workouts in all the major areas of fitness. The primary goals of a pre-season conditioning program (Table 2-1) are to establish a solid fitness base for skill development, to condition all of the major fitness areas, and to provide a high level of fitness which will be maintained through the rest of the year. During this time squads are working on both new skill development and camp preparation.

IN-SEASON

Cheerleading usually encompasses two athletic seasons (football and basketball) plus minor sports, pep rallies, spirit raising activities, community service, and competitions. Cheerleaders are **busy** during this time, therefore, the primary goal of an in-season conditioning program (Tables 2-2 and 2-3) is to maintain the fitness base established in the pre-season. The in-season program helps prevent overuse type injuries and provides us with the necessary physical condition to improve our skills year-round.

Considering the length of the season, there are a couple tips which will help you get productive workouts during the in-season part of the year. 1) Cheerleaders should be checked regularly for any signs of undue fatigue or symptoms of overtraining. An occasional full week of recovery is a good preventative measure in this regard. These short breaks also provide good opportunities to perform fitness evaluations. At this time you can determine if the program is actually maintaining the pre-season conditioning level that you worked so hard to attain, or if changes are needed. Special consideration of this problem should be given during the transition between sports, during the competition schedule and as cheerleading season comes to a close. 2) In addition to full days off, alternation of light, medium and heavy workout intensities during the in-season period is important to allow for recovery prior to games and other performances. Altering the intensity of workouts also gives the program variety which helps with motivation.

** Remember: The following tables are sample conditioning programs. Based on your current level of fitness and your fitness needs, fill in the best exercises that will help you reach your conditioning goals. Select exercises from those outlined in chapters 3-6 or use your own!

SAMPLE CONDITIONING PROGRAMS

Key to Abbreviations

Types of Conditioning	Workout duration		Workout intensity
	minimum	maximum	
flex - flexibility	10 minutes	30 minutes	L - light intensity
end - endurance	10 minutes	30 minutes	M - medium intensity
str/pow - strength/power	45 minutes	60 minutes	H - heavy intensity
ment - mental 10 minutes	30 minutes		

Table 2-1.

PRE-SEASON
Summer Program

Monday	Tuesday	Wednesday	Thursday	Friday	Saturday	Sunday
flex	flex	flex	flex	flex	flex	flex
str/pow	end	str/pow	end	str/pow	end	
	ment		ment		ment	

Table 2-2.

IN-SEASON
Fall Program

Monday	Tuesday	Wednesday	Thursday	Friday	Saturday	Sunday
flex	end-H	flex	end-M	flex		
str/pow-H	ment	str/pow-M	ment	str/pow-L		

Table 2-3.

IN-SEASON
Winter Program

Monday	Tuesday	Wednesday	Thursday	Friday	Saturday	Sunday
end-H	game	str/pow-M	end-M	game	str-pow-H	
ment		flex	ment	flex		

ENDURANCE
Chapter 3

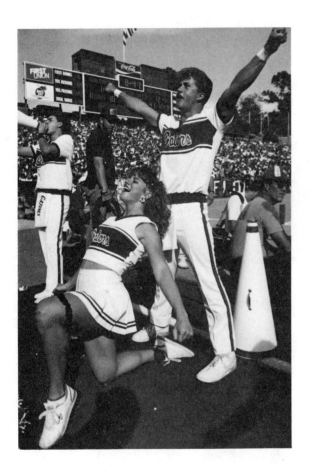

Any cheerleader who has ever tried to cheer through an entire game will understand the subject of this chapter! **Endurance is your capacity to sustain movement over a period of time.** Good endurance will enable you to have enough stamina and strength to engage in vigorous activity such as cheerleading. It also implies the soundness of body organs such as your heart and your lungs.

The two types of endurance are **muscular** and **respiratory/circulatory.** When you have good muscular endurance you can continue successive movements when the muscles or muscle group involved are used beyond "normal" activity. You are able to work over a longer period of time and the recovery rate of your muscles will be faster.

Recovery rate is the length of time it takes your muscles and cardiorespiratory system to return to their resting state after exercise. The more fit you are, the faster your recovery rate.

THE IMPORTANCE OF ENDURANCE TRAINING FOR CHEERLEADERS

Your ability to continuously perform jumps, tumbling, cheers, etc. without getting too tired is a result of good muscular and cardiorespiratory endurance. The combined function of the heart, lungs, and circulatory vessels is an important factor in peak performance. When your cardiorespiratory system fails to meet the demands of cheerleading your performance suffers.

YOUR BODY DURING AEROBIC WORKOUTS

During strenuous aerobic exercise, your body uses oxygen at a very high rate. If it is not delivered quickly enough or in sufficient quantities, your body develops an oxygen deficiency, eventually contributing to fatigue. Increasing your cardiorespiratory endurance can correct this by improving your body's capacity to take in and use oxygen. How does this happen?

YOUR CARDIORESPIRATORY SYSTEM

The heart's primary function during exercise is to deliver oxygenated blood to the cells and to remove metabolic byproducts. The amount of oxygen utilized by the body during maximum exercise for a particular period of time is referred to as **maximum oxygen intake.** Maximum oxygen uptake is therefore one of the best indicators of cardiorespiratory fitness. In order to increase your body's ability to use oxygen, endurance training is essential.

Your heart, lungs and circulatory vessels make up your cardiorespiratory system. The heart is

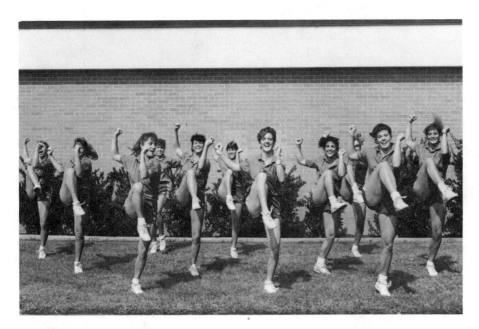

composed of four chambers: the left and right atria (upper chambers) and the left and right ventricles (lower chambers). Your heart is approximately the size of your fist and weighs under a pound. Blood travels from the right atrium into the right ventricle, leaving the heart through the pulmonary artery and moving into the lungs, where the blood then releases carbon dioxide and picks up more oxygen. The two pulmonary veins transport blood to the left atrium of the heart, into the left ventricle and then out the aorta, the main artery of the body, which branches to all parts of your anatomy.

Tiny blood vessels connecting the arteries with the veins are called capillaries. In these vessels, oxygen is released from the blood into the cells and carbon dioxide is removed from the tissues. The veins transport the cells and carbon dioxide-rich blood back to the right atrium by way of the inferior and superior vena cava, completing the cycle of blood flow.

> *"Our squad started an endurance training program last spring. We can tell a big difference in our energy level and we were wondering what changes have taken place to make us notice the increased energy level."*

ENERGY SYSTEMS

Your body has three energy systems. Two of these systems are **anaerobic, meaning without oxygen.** The third is the aerobic system. **Aerobic means with oxygen.** The first system, called ATP (adenosinetriphosphate), is the immediate form of muscular energy. ATP is stored in the muscles at rest. It is the initial system used for quick, short periods of time which last **less than 30 seconds.** Clapping, jumping, or performing a back handspring are all examples of ATP.

The body's second system is **anaerobic glycolysis.** This system is used when the activity is **between 30 seconds and three minutes.** An example would be performing a short dance routine. Your body's third energy system is the **aerobic or oxidative** system, used when a particular activity is **greater than three minutes.** Aerobic energy is needed for daily living functions in addition to the anaerobic energies. During prolonged activity you need the aerobic system to convert your food (fuel) into ATP's (energy).

Most activities require a blend of these specific systems. All three systems will contribute to any activity, however, one system will usually predominate.

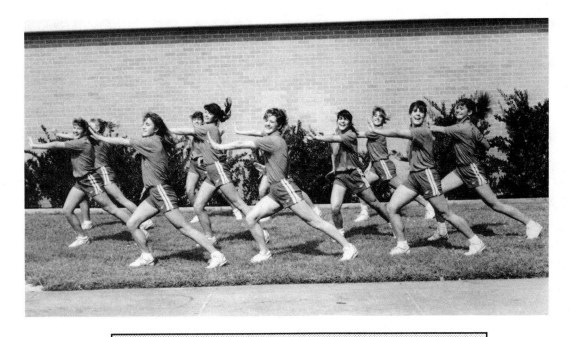

> *"No one on our squad has ever had any type of training in developing an endurance training program. What do we need to know to get started?"*

THE OVERLOAD PRINCIPLE

When your muscles or physiological systems (e.g., the cardiorespiratory system) are used beyond the point of comfort or are overloaded, strength and/or endurance is developed. The overload principle is more simply described as the F.I.T. principle.

Increasing the <u>Frequency</u> or the number of days a week, adding to the <u>I</u>ntensity level of the exercise (i.e., adding weights to an aerobic dance routine, increasing the tension on an exercise bicycle, adding more weight to your lifting routine), or increasing the length of <u>T</u>ime or duration of your work out per session will increase your level of fitness. Once you become comfortable with your routine and you want to improve your fitness level, a portion of the F.I.T. principle must be increased in order to maintain and overload.

If you plan to increase your level of endurance training by applying the F.I.T. principle, use only one part of the principle at a time. Do not try and reach your goal too quickly; progress slowly. Allow your body to adapt to the increased training level a little at a time. An example of this would be to increase the tension on your exercise bicycle and maintain that new level of intensity for weeks four through six of your twelve-week program. Then, weeks seven through ten, increase the length of your workout three to four minutes at the level of intensity reached in weeks four through six. You have now increased your overload twice by using two parts of the F.I.T. principle, and having done so gradually, there is less strain on the body.

METHODS OF ENDURANCE TRAINING

> *"Are there different types of training? If so, what do we need to know about them in order to figure out the best workout for our squad?"*

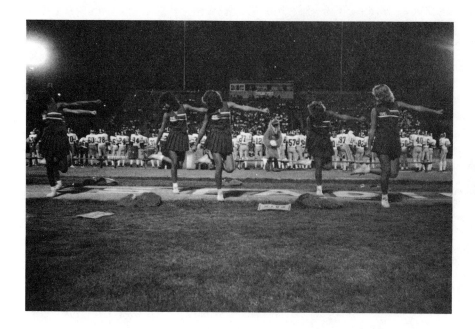

Continuous or discontinuous aerobic training may be used to improve cardiorespiratory endurance. Continuous methods would include jogging, running long, slow distances or continuous lap swimming. Discontinuous methods include Fartlek training, interval training and circuit weight training. A further explanation of circuit weight training can be found in chapter five.

CONTINUOUS TRAINING

Non-stop exercise at low to moderate intensity levels is considered continuous training. The most popular type of continuous training is long, slow distance running or jogging. Being able to maintain the appropriate intensity level (i.e., 70 percent maximum heart rate) is an advantage of the steady-paced exercise. In addition, low to moderate intensity lev-

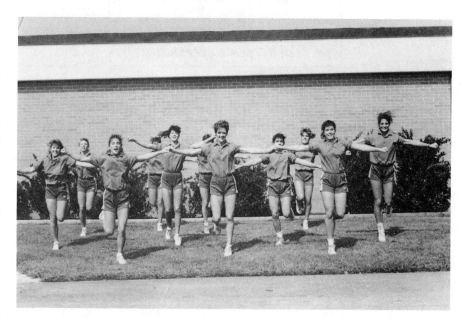

els are safer, more comfortable and better suited for cheerleaders just starting an aerobic conditioning program. The drop-out rate in high intensity interval training programs has been reported to be twice that of a continuous jogging program.

INTERVAL (DISCONTINUOUS) TRAINING

A workout program of exercises interspersed with rest periods is considered interval training. The exercise intensity and total amount of work performed can be greater than that of continuous training since rest periods are included in this type of training. The rest periods give you some degree of recovery, allowing you to put greater energy into your next exercise. You would also be able to increase the number or the duration of your exercises.

Let's demonstrate interval training using swimming. You would swim one length of the pool in 40-50 seconds, then rest one and a half to two minutes (keeping your body in motion).
Sets: 8 x 50 yards
Total distance: 400 yards
Time: 40-50 seconds per set
Rest period: 1 1/2 - 2 minutes between sets
By increasing the intensity of the exercise, decreasing the duration of the rest period between intervals or increasing the number of exercise intervals per workout, you are applying the overload principle. Interval training is recommended for cheerleaders who are able to tolerate moderate to high intensity exercise for short periods of time.

"FARTLEK TRAINING METHOD"

An adaptation of interval training is the Fartlek training method. This involves alternate fast and slow running over natural terrain. The rest period is not timed, but rather is based on how you feel during exercise. The duration of exercise in Fartlek training is usually 30-45 minutes. Use this type of training to add variety and enjoyment to your aerobic workout.

EXERCISE INTENSITY

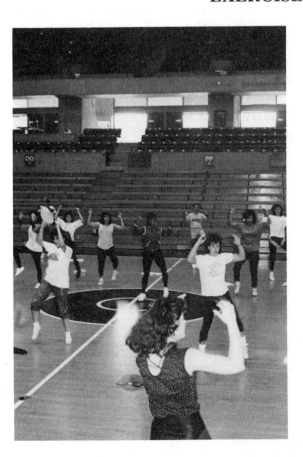

"Should our squad aerobic workout be exactly the same?
How can each of us tell if you are exercising hard enough
to get any aerobic benefit?"

Exercising with the **proper intensity** is the key to getting results. You need to work out with enough intensity to stress your cardiorespiratory system without putting too much strain on it. Since intensity of exercise is not always outwardly visible, how do you know if you are exercising too hard, not hard enough or just right?

Once you begin your program, you can check the intensity of your workout by **monitoring your heart rate** (see below). This simple process includes determining your "training pulse zone" (what your heart rate should be while you are exercising), then checking your heart rate while you exercise to make sure your heart rate is within your zone. Your "training pulse zone" is the number of heartbeats per minute that you need to reach while exercising in order to burn the most calories and achieve an optimal level of fitness. It's simple to figure out using this easy mathematical formula based on your age. (See page 22)

Instructions for Determining Your Training Pulse Zone.
1) Subtract your age from 220.
2) Multiply this figure by .7 to find the lowest end of your training zone.
3) Multiply 220 minus your age by .8 to find your upper limit.

If your heart rate is not where it should be, you can adjust your routine accordingly. The intensity of exercise is expressed as a percentage of the cardiorespiratory's aerobic capacity. This is usually 50 to 80 percent of the maximum oxygen uptake or 60 to 90 percent of maximum heart rate reserve.

Monitor your heart rate once before exercising, at least twice during and once after your workout so you will be constantly aware of your heart rate. Checking your heart rate before exercise lets you know your **resting heart rate.** Approximately three to four minutes into your routine, take your heart rate again and do so every four to five minutes throughout the exercise and cool down portion of your routine. Once you become familiar with this process, you will know your exercise intensity level and heart rate checks can be less frequent.

INSTRUCTIONS FOR TAKING YOUR HEART RATE:

1) Use your index and/or second finger to locate your pulse. Your exercising heart rate can be taken at the radial artery in your wrist or the carotid artery in the neck.
2) Count the number of beats you get for 10 seconds.
3) Multiply by six to get the approximate number of beats per minute.
4) This number should fall in the target heart rate zone.

CHOOSING YOUR AEROBIC EXERCISE

A number of endurance exercises are described in this chapter; keeping facilities and equipment in mind, select the workout that you will enjoy most. Use a combination of aerobic exercises or change the type of exercise after each twelve to sixteen week program for added variety.

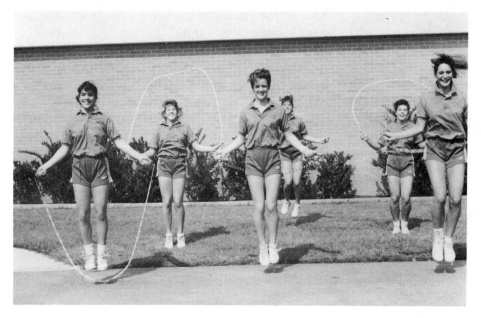

JOGGING

Jogging is one of the most widespread and popular forms of exercise. Many people use it as their only form of workout. Medical opinions differ as to the value and risk of jogging, but everyone agrees that it should be taken easily at first, especially for those who are overweight or unaccustomed to exercise.

Rather than plunge into a jogging program, you may want to start by walking, then alternate

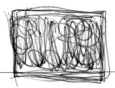

between walking and jogging for the first four weeks before attempting to jog your desired distance. A good test of the appropriate intensity level is to be able to jog and have enough energy and breath left to talk with someone next to you. If this is too difficult, you need to go back to alternating walking and jogging, decreasing the walking time until conversation becomes easy for you at jogging pace.

> *"No one on our squad likes to jog. What other types of aerobic exercise could we use for endurance training?"*

JUMP ROPE

What a great squad workout this is. In addition to being a physical challenge full of variety and creativity, jumping rope is excellent stimulation for your cardiorespiratory system and a good way to improve coordination.

The special advantages of rope skipping include shorter workouts! Because it is such a strenuous exercise, the time necessary for conditioning gains is shorter (20 minutes minimum) than other aerobics. Less of a strain is put on your legs and feet than in running. You don't have to deal with the weather and it is inexpensive, requiring little space or equipment.

Don't try to skip rope too fast. Concentrate on consistency. Increase your workout time week by week and gradually increase the pace until you find the one that will allow you to skip rope your desired time without having to rest. If you reach the point of breathlessness (where you can't pass the Talk Test) or find that your exercising heart rate is too high, relax by walking until you catch your breath.

SWIMMING

If a pool is available to you, swimming is a great workout! The water has a cushioning effect and there is no contact with the ground. Swimming is an excellent method of rehabilitation therapy for cheerleaders who have been injured or suffer from arthritis or tendonitis. Water provides the resistance needed to regain strength without direct impact and its cushioning effect may act to massage painful joints or sore areas.

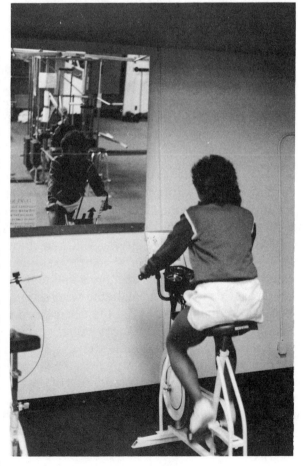

Swimming is a relatively injury free sport as long as proper warm-up and cool down exercises are followed. A muscle strain in the back or shoulder area is the common exception to this rule and is usually the result of over-training.

You are going to need a high degree of cardiorespiratory endurance in swimming as well as strength in your ams, shoulders and abdomen. In addition, the back and breast strokes require strong legs; a strong back is also needed for the breast stroke. Good joint flexibility is needed for swimming, especially in the knee and shoulder areas.

CYCLING

Cycling is a fantastic stamina builder. It demands great heart and lung endurance, as well as

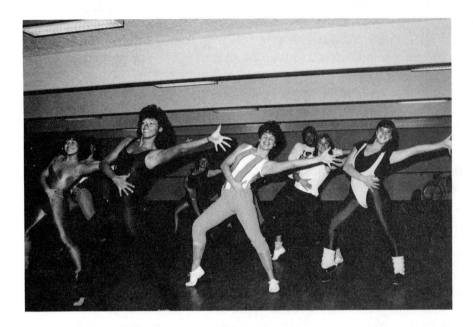

muscular endurance in the lower body and legs. Being a non-weight bearing exercise, cycling provides less chance of injury to your lower body. If you cannot participate in jogging or aerobic dance due to lower back or leg problems, cycling is highly recommended.

AEROBIC DANCE

Aerobic dance is a combination of rhythmic movements and simple dance steps to music to improve and maintain cardiorespiratory fitness. Many cheerleading squads incorporate this type of exercise in their normal practice because, with the right music and routine, it can also be a lot of fun! Since the type of instruction you can receive is widely varied (and can often be too difficult for beginners), be sure to follow a quality workout that has been developed by a professional.

The target heart rate is harder to maintain in aerobic dance than in other aerobics because of the wide variety of steps and movement directions used, as well as the different levels of intensity in which a step can be performed. Aerobic dance is also more prone to producing injury due to the direct impact to the feet and legs. A low impact class is great for beginners, as well as for those with joint or bone problems.

BENEFITS OF CARDIORESPIRATORY TRAINING

A number of physiological and anatomical chapters can result with cardiorespiratory training. A moderate increase in the heart size is a normal response to exercise training. The athlete's "enlarged" muscular heart is capable of generating a larger stroke volume due to forceful systolic ejections which result in greater ventrical emptying. Cardiorespiratory training also results in reduction of the heart rate for the same level of work or an increased work output at the same heart rate.

Maximal oxygen uptake decreases and percent body fat increases with age. There is evidence to suggest that this trend can be altered with endurance training. Cardiorespiratory training is essential in body fat reduction as oxygen is necessary for the fat burning process. Oxygen consumption is increased during cardiorespiratory exercise. This increased metabolic rate slowly decreases back to normal, taking up to several hours after exercise, depending on its intensity level. Lower blood pressure and a decreased rate of breathing are also the result of endurance training.

Endurance training is a necessary part of a total fitness program and is a must for cheerleaders. Peak performance in cheerleading will only be possible once you are aerobically fit. Develop your endurance and you will not only look great, you will feel great—all the way through the fourth quarter!

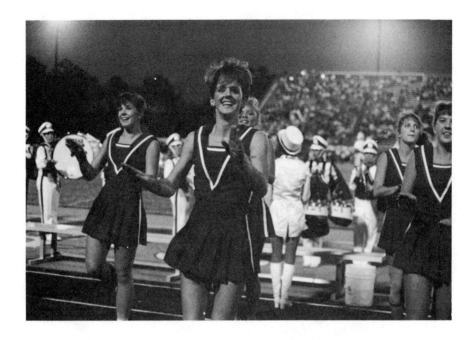

SAMPLE AEROBIC PROGRAMS

The following are sample aerobic exercise programs for beginning, intermediate and advanced levels. The muscle groups listed for a particular exercise are those that are primary to the exercise. Be sure to do the warmups and proper stretching before the exercise. A complete endurance training program should include a warm-up, an aerobic training period, the cool-down, and a recommended strength conditioning period. As you plan your exercise program, keep in mind the following:

1. **Frequency of training** — 3-5 days a week.
2. **Intensity of training** — 60-90 percent of the maximum heart rate reserve.
3. **Duration of training** — 20-60 minutes of continuous aerobic activity. (Duration is dependent on the intensity of your activity. Lower intensity activity should be conducted over a longer period of time. Lower to moderate intensity activity of longer duration is recommended for the non-athletic individual because of the potential hazards and complicated problems associated with high intensity activity.)
4. **Mode of activity** — Any activity using large muscle groups which can be maintained continuously and is rhythmic in nature. Such activities include walking, jogging, running, swimming, bicycling, rowing, cross-country skiing, jumping rope and aerobic dance.

WALKING/JOGGING
Beginning

Primary Muscles	Week(s)	Distance Miles	Time
Hamstrings	1 & 2	1.0	13:30-15:00
Quadriceps	3 & 4	1.0	13:00-14:00
Calves	5 & 6	1.0	12:45-13:45
Heart	7 & 8	1.0 - 1.5	11:45-21:30
	9 & 10	1.0 - 1.5	11:00-21:00
	11 & 12	1.0 - 1.5	10:30-20:30

Intermediate

	Week(s)	Distance Miles	Time
	1 & 2	1.5 - 2.0	17:30-27:30
	3 & 4	2.0	17:00-27:00
	5 & 6	2.0	16:30-26:30
	7 & 8	2.5 - 3.0	23:00-40:00
	9 & 10	2.5 - 3.0	22:30-39:30
	11 & 12	3.0	24:00-39:00

Advanced

	Week(s)	Distance Miles	Time
	1 & 2	3.0	up to 32:30
	3 & 4	3.0 - 3.5	up to 31:30
	5 & 6	3.0 - 3.5	up to 29:45
	7 & 8	3.5	up to 28:00
	9 & 10	3.5	up to 27:30
	11 & 12	2.5 - 4.0	up to 32:00

SWIMMING
Beginning
(use an additional 50 yard warm-up swim)

Primary Muscles	Week(s)	Sets	Total Distance
Deltoids	1 - 2	4 x 25 & 2 x 50	200 yards
Trapezius	3 - 4	6 x 25 & 2 x 50	250 yards
Pectoral	5 - 7	3 x 50 & 2 x 75	300 yards
Latisimus Dorsi	8 - 9	5 x 75	375 yards
Hamstrings	10 - 12	3 x 75 & 2 x 100	425 yards
Quadriceps Heart			

Intermediate
(use an additional 75-125 year warm-up swim)

1 - 4	4 x75 & 2 x 100	500 yards
5 - 8	3 x 75 & 3 x 125	600 yards
9 - 12	3 x 75 & 3 x 150	675 yards

Advanced
(use an additional 150-200 yard warm-up swim)

1 - 3	2 x 75 & 4 x 150	750 yards
4 - 6	3 x 100 & 3 x 175	835 yards
7 - 9	2 x 150 & 3 x 200	900 yards
10 - 12	3 x 150 & 3 x 200	1050 yards

AEROBIC DANCE

Aerobic dance classes range from low impact to high intensity levels and include an extremely wide variety of formats. Suggested recommendations for selecting an aerobic dance class/program have been described previously in this chapter.

CYCLING
Beginning

Main Muscle Groups	Weeks	Distance Miles	Time Minutes
Quadriceps	1 - 2	4.0	20:00
Hamstrings	3 - 4	4.25	20:00
Calves	5 - 6	4.50	20:00
Heart	7 - 8	4.75	20:00
	9 - 10	5.00	20:00
	11 - 12	5.00	20:00

Intermediate

	Weeks	Distance Miles	Time Minutes
	1 - 3	5.25	20:00
	4 - 6	5.50	20:00
	7 - 9	5.75	20:00
	10-12	6.00	20:00

CYCLING (PROGRESSIVE-STATIONARY)

Vigorous Cycling	Slow Cycling	Load	Approximate Distance Of Vigorous Cycling
1 mile or 5 min (12 mph cycling speed)	1/4 mile or 2 min	Start 2/5 sets; then in each succeeding workout, add a set until you can do 8 sets	5-8 miles
1 mile or 4 min (15 mph cycling speed)	1/4 mile or 2 min	Start w/5 sets; then in each succeeding workout add a set until you can do 10 sets	5-10 miles
1 1/2 mile or 6 min (15 mph cycling speed)	1/3 mile or 3 min	Start w/4 sets; then in each succeeding workout add a set until you can do 10 sets	6-15 miles
2 miles or 8 min (15 mph cycling speed)	1/3 mile or 3 min	Start w/4 sets; then in each succeding workout add a set until you can do 10 sets.	10-20 miles
10-20 miles or 40 min to 1 /2/3 hrs of continuous cycling 12-15 mph cycling speed	Every 5 miles you may wish to cycle for a mile at a reduced speed.		

JUMPING ROPE

	THR	FREQUENCY	DURATION
Jump for 60 seconds and then rest for 60 seconds. Repeat six to eight times (4-10 minutes)	60%	3 days	2-4 weeks
Jump for 90 seconds and then rest for 30 seconds. Repeat four to eight times (8-12 minutes)	70%	3 days	2-4 weeks
Jump for 2 minutes and then rest for 30 seconds. Repeat four to eight times (10-25 minutes)	70%	3-5 days	2-4 weeks
Jump for 4 minutes and then rest for 30 seconds. Repeat four to eight times. (15-30 minutes)	70%	3-5 days	2-4 weeks
Jump for 8 minutes and then rest for 30 seconds. Repeat one to two times. (15-30 minutes)	70%	3-5 days	2-4 weeks
Jump for 10 minutes and then rest for 2 to 3 minutes. Repeat one to two times. (30 minutes)	70%	3-5 days	2-4 weeks

STRENGTH AND POWER TRAINING
Chapter Four

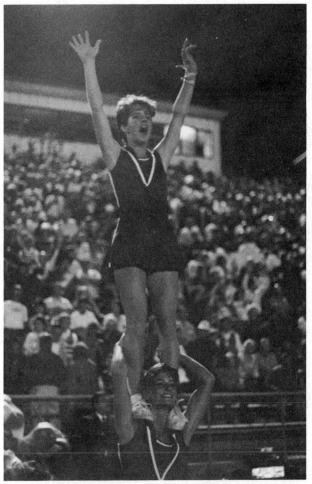

Would you like to reduce your chances of injury in all the different cheering skills you perform? Do you know of any cheerleaders who need to increase the height of their jumps? Is your squad's stunt performance limited due to a lack of strength? Do you think there are many cheerleaders around who would love to be able to perform excellent gymnastics? If you are answering "YES!" to any of these important questions, then this chapter on Strength and Power training is for YOU! Nothing will replace physical cheerleading practices, however, if you are serious about improving your skills, incorporating a strength and power training program is an extremely beneficial use of your squad practice time!

The strength and power training best for you depends on many factors including the type of squad you are or hope to be a member of (co-ed, collegiate, high school, junior high), and the facilities available to you (at school, in your home, in local gyms, etc.). Let's start by examining the need for strength and power development, how it actually affects your cheerleading performance, and then plan a workout based on available facilities, personal level of fitness and athletic goals.

HOW TO USE THIS CHAPTER

You'll soon notice this chapter is detailed and very possibly, all the information will not be relevant to your current level of athletic achievement. The physiological explanations have been included to give cheerleaders and coaches the opportunity to **completely understand** the cheerleader body and athletic potential. Since your goals will vary from the next reader, use as much or little of this chapter as you need. The important point is to determine your athletic needs!

Your squad will outline many team goals, but **only you can determine what degree of athletic excellence you plan to achieve!** Naturally, junior high cheerleader goals differ from collegiate cheerleader goals. One thing we all have in common is the desire to develop our athletic ability, thus all cheerleaders need to develop some degree of strength and power. The first step is to understand **why**. Before we learn actual exercises, let's understand some basic definitions, principles and concepts concerned with strength and power training.

PHYSIOLOGY OF MUSCLE

The three principle components of muscle function which can be improved through training to enhance your cheerleading performance are **strength**, **power** and **muscular** endurance.

"Even though my squad understands proper technique for performing partner stunts, our bases often 'walk' with their stunts instead of remaining stable. Does this have to do with strength?"

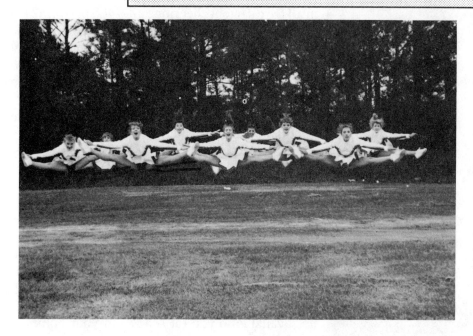

STRENGTH

Although definitions vary, we will define strength as the amount of force that can be developed in a static (no movement) contraction (Atha, 1981). This type of strength is seen in a partner stunt where there is no visible movement.

"No matter how hard I try, my jumps are always low. I practice and practice but I just can't seem to get high up in the air."

POWER

Power can be viewed as strength (force) x velocity, which includes the component of movement or speed. Be sure to understand how power differs from strength because **power is vital to your skill development!** Improve your power output and your cheerleading abilities will greatly increase. Power training will enable you to exert greater amounts of force in a shorter period of time, thereby leading to in-

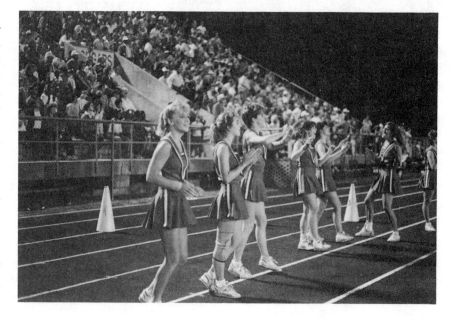

creases in vertical jump as well as making your stunts and tumbling much easier.

> *"I coach a squad that cheers with lots of energy until the fourth quarter rolls around. Then, they fall apart, as if they are so tired they can't even perform a shoulder stand safely."*

MUSCULAR ENDURANCE

The third fundamental property of muscle function following strength and power is muscular endurance. Increasing your **muscular endurance**, through proper training will help **delay fatigue**. Imagine how extra muscular endurance will improve your performance and, more importantly, the safety element of each skill. If you are overly tired, safety should be your primary concern when considering the performance of gymnastics, stunts and pyramids. Your muscular endurance is quite evident as the end of a game draws near and peak physical condition in this area is vital to a good cheering squad.

PHYSIOLOGICAL BENEFITS OF STRENGTH AND POWER TRAINING

How do increases in strength and power take place? Physiological changes from strength and power training take place in three major areas — neural (nervous system), muscular, and biochemical.

NEURAL (NERVOUS SYSTEM)

The first increases in your strength level (up to three weeks) are mainly due to neural effects. Mastering the movement pattern seems to increase the efficiency of muscle activity, eliciting strength without an increase in muscle fiber size, or hypertrophy (Hakikinen and Komi, 1983).

MUSCULAR

The two types of muscular changes that will help you develop power are **hypertrophy** and **plyometrics**. To get the benefits of both aspects of power, you must train both systems. Hypertrophy has to do with increasing the size of your muscles and is developed through weight training. There is a direct connection between the cross-sectional area (CSA) of a muscle fiber and the maximum force produced. Therefore a larger muscle (i.e. one with a greater CSA) will be able to produce greater amounts of force.

Plyometric jump training involves storing and using elastic energy. When you punch off the ground for a jump, upon landing, elastic energy is stored in your quadriceps, gluteal, and calf muscles. As you begin to push off the ground for your jump, this stored elastic energy is released and utilized allowing you to jump higher than if you did a vertical jump starting from a static position with bent knees. **Plyometric training will increase the storage and utilization of elastic energy, ultimately increasing the height of your vertical jump or your punch off the ground during a tumbling pass.**

BIOCHEMICAL

Several biochemical changes will occur in your muscles as you train. The fuels required to produce energy for your muscles to contract become more plentiful and are used more effectively with increased enzyme levels. The particular fuels and enzymes your body produces will depend upon the type of training method you use. For example, power training will increase your muscles' ability to contract more quickly and with greater force; whereas, strength training will increase your muscles' ability to maintain a static contraction. These biochemical changes directly apply to your ability to perform better jumps, tumbling passes and stunts as well as recover faster between performing these skills.

MUSCLE MASS AND BODY COMPOSITION

Male cheerleaders want to increase the size of their muscles; however, female cheerleaders are usually afraid that a strength and power workout will leave them with huge, bulky muscles. Since **the idea of females "bulking up" is a major misconception**, let's take a closer look. The cause of muscle mass differences in males and females for the most part is hormonal. Testosterone is a greater stimulator for protein synthesis (resulting in muscle growth) than is estrogen. The differences in muscle mass, and therefore strength, are primarily due to the high levels of testosterone produced by males. Females, on the other hand, produce very little testosterone and high levels of estrogen.

If you are a female cheerleader, rest assured that strength and power training will not put enormous muscles on your figure. You will, however, have a **change in body composition** (see Chapter Seven), gaining some muscle and losing fat. When this occurs, at the same scale weight, you will **look leaner** because per unit volume muscle, having a greater density, weighs more than fat. If you are still convinced you will "bulk up" if you get in the weight room, have your testosterone levels checked by a physician.

TRAINING PRINCIPLES

OVERLOAD PRINCIPLE

The three key principles of S/P training are "Overload," "Specificity" and "Reversibility." The **Overload Principle** requires muscles to be overloaded beyond an implied threshold point in order for change to take place. Increase weight progressively throughout the course of your program in order to keep the overload above this threshold.

It is important to note that high school and college cheerleaders should begin with their own body weight (if they have not trained before) and train up to 30 percent of the body weight. The overload principle of resistance other than body weight is **not recommended for cheerleaders under 13 to 14 years of age** because of the chance of injury due to insufficient growth plate development.

SPECIFICITY PRINCIPLE

The **Specificity Principle** simply means you must keep your exercises similar to the demands of cheerleading activity. The closer you mimic cheerleading movement in your workout, the greater the resulting benefits will improve your skill performance.

REVERSIBILITY PRINCIPLE.

The final principle is Reversibility. If you don't use it, you lose it! Your muscles adjust to less use so if you miss a workout or take a week off, you will begin to lose the training effect. As a general guideline, **train three times per week with a day of rest in between workouts for recovery.**

> **Table 4-1.**
> Isometric: Weight = Muscle Force = no movement
> Concentric: Weight < Muscle Force = muscle shortening
> Eccentric: Weight > Muscle Force = muscle lengthening

MUSCLE CONTRACTIONS

Determining your training technique begins by discussing muscle contractions, usually referred to as **isometric, concentric or eccentric** (Table 4-1). An isometric contraction is static. No visible movement occurs because the load of the weight being lifted is equal to the force produced internally by the muscle. This is often demonstrated in partner stunts. The drawback associated with isometric training is that it increases your strength only at specific joint angles of your training. Since nearly all athletic activities involve movement, your weight training sessions should attempt copying that movement.

Concentric contraction refers to a shortening contraction of the muscle, where the weight is less than the internal force exerted by muscle. For example, in a bicep curl, your biceps shorten while you are lifting the weight. An **eccentric** contraction refers to a controlled lengthening of the muscle where the weight is greater than the force exerted by the muscle. For example, in a bicep curl, your biceps lengthen while you are lowering the weight.

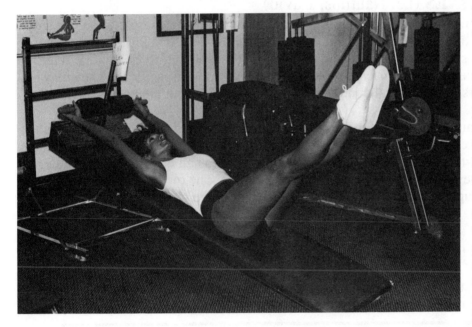

DYNAMIC TRAINING

Most cheerleading movement is not static; instead it is **dynamic** (energy or physical force in motion) and this includes both concentric and eccentric muscle activity. You will benefit the most from a dynamic training program. Include either free weight training, variable resistance training (i.e. Nautilus), accommodating resistance training (i.e. Cybex), plyometric training and/or circuit training depending on your specific needs.

TYPES OF TRAINING

CIRCUIT TRAINING AND NON-WEIGHT BEARING EXERCISES

Cheerleaders who have no prior training experience should begin training with non-weight bearing exercise. This means using your body weight only, ie. sit-ups, push-ups, dips, etc. Most exercises outlined later in this chapter have both weight bearing and non-weight bearing variations.

A great way to begin your workout for the first 3-6 weeks of training is circuit training (see guideline, page 37). It is easy to organize and will allow your squad to work out efficiently together. Cheerleaders need a certain amount of endurance to perform at their best as the end of the game draws near and fatigue begins to set in. However, many cheerleading movements are explosive, and to enhance performance, power development must be emphasized as the season approaches.

PLYOMETRIC POWER DEVELOPMENT

For the most power development, train dynamically at the appropriate speed and include plyometric training as a part of your workout. Plyometric exercises will help you "explode" with power in your jumps, tumbling, stunts, and so on. Include various hopping and bounding on flat surfaces, jump squats and depth jump sequences, and double leg hops lateral and forward.

FREE WEIGHTS (Barbells and Dumbbells)

Specificity is probably most closely followed when you use free weight. This type of training allows you to actively accelerate and more effectively maintain your power output; therefore, you will more effectively stress the components of your neuromuscular system that are responsible for power. Adjusting your movement speed to leverage changes in your body is called **Compensatory Acceleration.** With free weights, you can simulate cheering movement and the higher speeds to a great extent.

RESISTANCE MACHINES (i.e. Nautilus, David)

Variable resistance machines, such as Nautilus, are better able to stress a muscle to its capacity through the full range of motion. However, they fail to emphasize balance. In addition, they cannot withstand the rigors of high speed training and tend, unlike sport movement, to isolate one muscle group at a time. Thus, variable resistance machines seem to defy the Law of Specificity. They may be used effectively by beginners in the general conditioning part of training, but are not recommended for advanced cheerleaders.

An accommodating resistance machine, such as Cybex, is a device that can produce a load (weight) equal in size to that generated by the muscle group but opposite in direction. Since the speed of movement remains constant throughout the exercise, it is referred to as an **isokinetic contraction**. Thus, muscle and load torques are equal and speed remains the same. The main benefit of isokinetic training is that a muscle group can be stressed maximally throughout the range of motion.

TRAINING SAFETY

To keep potential injuries from occurring and to maximize your workout, always remain serious about each exercise you and fellow squad members are performing. This is no time for "horsing around." Train hard, like the athletes cheerleaders have become (not like the stereotype of old!). When you are in the weight room, it is necessary to take the following precautions:

> 1. Make sure you train with an organized program.
> 2. If you don't know proper procedure, ask; if there is no one to ask, don't do it.
> 3. Wear proper shoes (no thongs or sandals).
> 4. Do not train alone. Work out with a partner.
> 5. Wear a lifting belt when recommended.
> 6. Load and unload the bar evenly.
> 7. Increase weight gradually, 10 percent at the most over one lifting session.
> 8. Always warm up properly and warm down to finish.
> 9. Avoid over-training.

DEVELOPING YOUR YEAR-ROUND WORKOUT

There are different ways you can set up your training program; however, remember that a cheerleader's season lasts all year! In order to perform at your peak year-round, it is a wise idea to begin your program following tryouts and continue your plan through basketball season. You can divide the year into three seasons: Pre-Season, In-Season, and the Transition Phases.

It goes without saying **you want results without wasting time and energy on non-productive workouts.** As you organize your program, remember you will be wasting time and energy if you do the exact same exercises in the same manner all year long! Instead, carefully plan the intensity, frequency and duration of your workout so you will get the results you are working for!

INTENSITY (WEIGHT) AND VOLUME (REPITITIONS)

The intensity and volume of your year-round training program should be designed so that you are in peak physical condition during the In-Season. Divide your Pre-Season into two parts: a General Conditioning, where circuit training may be done for 3-6 weeks, and a Specific Conditioning, where weight training sessions are more specific to cheerleading movements. Ideally, your Pre-Season program should last at least 16 weeks (May-August) in order for you to perform at a high level during the entire In-Season (beginning in September).

It is best to have beginning cheerleaders use their own body weight initially. You will progress up to 25 to 30 percent of your body weight. When a weight is a challenge to lift but you are not struggling, this is a good weight to use. Increase the weight or the number of repetitions once the current weight/reps are no longer a challenge. Remember, every person is different, so do not set standard weights for your entire squad.

DURATION (TIME)

How long should each workout last? You must first ask yourself how much time do you have? Training sessions depend on many factors, including the time of year, your skill level and facilities. You are much busier during the In-Season once school begins, so you should plan to train harder during the Pre-Season (May-August), then maintain your strength in the fall and winter.

In-Season workouts should ideally last a minimum of 45 minutes; however, remember consistent workout is the key. So even if you can only devote 20 to 30 minutes to training, do it! During the pre-season, you should train longer (no longer than an hour and a half). For example, your Pre-Season Program may take an hour, where as the In-Season program may only be 45 minutes. You will have to be the judge of the time you can devote to strength and power training.

FREQUENCY

How Often Should You Train Each Week? The frequency of your workout during your Pre-Season will be different than in your In-Season and depends on your goals and time available to train. You must decide for yourself what results you are looking for, then you can determine how much time to devote to strength and power development. **Remember, build up strength during your Pre-Season; maintain strength throughout the year.**

WORKOUT FREQUENCY
PRE-SEASON AND TRANSITIONS

**Minimal:	2 x per week, Tues/Thurs
**Ideal:	3 x per week, 1-2 day(s) of rest between sessions
	For example: Mon/Wed/Fri
**Split Routine:	4 x per week
For example:	Mon/Thurs = Upper Body Exercises
	Tues/Fri = Lower body Exercises
**Split Routine:	6 x per week
	For example: Mon/Wed/Fri = Upper Body Exercises
	Tues/Thurs/Sat = Lower Body Exercises

IN-SEASON

**Maintenance Phase - 2 x per week	
For example:	Monday = Heavy Day
	Wednesday = Medium Day
	Game on Friday or Saturday

TRANSITION PHASE OF TRAINING

The Transition Phase is the time period after the In-Season is over and before the next Pre-Season begins. The entire month of April would be the transition phase for most cheerleaders. This is a time of "Active Rest," a time to get out of the weight room and cheerleading modes. It is extremely important to be active physically in other ways so you won't lose all that you worked so hard to obtain! Your activities should be fun, yet physically stressing, such as: cycling, racquetball, swimming, basketball, soccer, etc. It is important to start the next cheerleading season refreshed both mentally and physically!

OVERTRAINING (VARIATION AND RECOVERY)

Every cheerleader on your squad should be aware of the possibility of "overtraining" and the negative effects this can have on your performance. If the following signs and symptoms of the "Overtraining State" are affecting you, it is suggested to give yourself three days to one week completely off from physical training. Then only do two sets of each exercise, by substituting different exercises that work the same muscles. **The most obvious result of overtraining is a decrease in your working capacity and performance.**

Implementing a strength and power program into your cheerleading workout has an incredible potential of improving your performance! Your jumps will be higher, your stunts will be more solid, your tumbling will be quicker and stronger, the list is endless. With the commitment and hours of hard work behind you, watch your self-confidence rise! Strengthening the body properly will help prevent injuries and can improve your overall health. Remember, some training is better than none. Just educate yourself, set your goals and go for it!

PRE SEASON PART ONE
Beginning Conditioning: General Conditioning Circuit Training
May (4 weeks) - 3 times per week

The following Circuit Training Workout is suggested for your squad to begin training. During your first week, complete two sets of all 10 exercises each workout day. By your second week, you should be able to complete 3 sets each session and you will continue this routine during the third and fourth week. Perform each repetition as fast as possible, keeping the proper form. No rest should be taken in between exercise stations. Only rest 60 seconds between your sets. Use the figure numbers to refer to the exercise photographs and descriptions at the end of the chapter.

NOTE: The following is a sample workout. Feel free to substitute exercises that have the same training effect.

Exercise station		Figure	Number of Repetitions
1.	squat thrusts	4-19	10-15
2.	push ups	4-11	10-20
3.	walking lunges	4-25	16-20 steps
4.	bent over rows	4-6	10-20
5.	free hand squat jumps	4-27	10-20
6.	upright rows	4-7	10-20
7.	bent-knee sit ups	4-2	15-25
8.	bench or bar dips	4-9	15-25
9.	back extensions on floor	4-3	10-20
10.	jump rope (high knees)	4-20	40-60 jumps

PRE-SEASON PART TWO
WEIGHT TRAINING FOR BEGINNERS
June - August (12 weeks) - 3 times per week (Mon/Wed/Fri)
60-90 minutes (ideally)

After completing the pre-season part one workout, you are ready to begin Part Two: power development in the weight room. If you have never lifted free weights before, or have limited experience, start with the Beginning Program. If you are an experienced lifter you may begin with the Intermediate Program. **Every cheerleader should complete at least one year of the Intermediate Program before moving on to the Advanced program.** Be sure to warm up before you work out with a five-minute jog or similar aerobic exercise and stretch out (flexibility) after each lifting session.

The beginning program is designed for cheerleaders who have little or no experience lifting weights to improve body strength and conditioning level, (most cheerleaders fall into this category). Train 12 weeks on this program before moving on to the intermediate program.

Exercise	Figure	Major Muscle Group(s)	Sets x Number of Repetitions
1. Bench Press	4-11	Pectorals, Anterior Deltoids - Triceps	3 x 8
2. Lat Pull-Downs	4-5	Latissimus Dorsi	3 x 8
3. Seated Military Press	4-12	Deltoids, Trapezius, Triceps	3 x 8
4. Dips	4-9	Triceps, Anterior Deltoids, Pectorals	3 x max.
5. Barbell Curls	4-8	Biceps	3 x 8
6. Free Hand Squat	4-26	Biceps	3 x 8
7. Free Hand Jump Squat	4-27	Same as 6.	3 x 8
8. Lunges	4-25	Same as 6.	3 x 16 steps
9. Ab/Adduction	4-17	Hip Ab/Adductors	3 x 10 each
10. Leg Extension	4-24	Quadriceps	3 x 10
11. Leg Curl	4-25	Hamstrings	3 x 10
12. Calf Raises	4-30	Gastrocnemius, Soleus, Plantaris	3 x 10
13. Abdominal Series	4-2	Rectus Abdominis	2 x 10 each
14. Back Extensions	4-3	Erector Spinae	2 x 10

IN-SEASON PROGRAM
(Beginning in SEPTEMBER or OCTOBER)
BEGINNING PROGRAM

Continue your same weight training program, however, cut down to two lifting sessions per week (Mon/Wed).

Intermediate and Advanced Programs (2 x per week)

Monday	=	HEAVY DAY	(4 x 4 on Primary Lifts)
			(Approx. 80-85% 1 Repetition Maximum)
Wednesday	=	MEDIUM DAY	(3-4 x 6 on Primary Lifts)
			(Approx. 70-75% 1 RM)

Friday or Saturday . . . PERFORM!

INTERMEDIATE PROGRAM

The intermediate program is designed for cheerleaders who are experienced free weight lifters. Be sure to consult with a Strength Coach to learn the proper form on the Push Press and Squat exercises. **Always** wear a lifting belt and have proper spotting on these exercises. See page 40 for the cycling of events and repetitions on the Primary Lifts.

Exercise	Figure	Major Muscle Group(s)	Sets x Number of Repetitions
1. Push Press	4-21	Gluteal Muscles, Quadriceps, Upper Hamstrings, Gastrocnemius, Deltoids, Trapezius, Triceps	4 x 8**
2. Bench Press	4-11	Pectorals, Anterior Deltoids, Triceps	4 x 8**
3. Back Squat	4-26	Gluteal Muscles, Quadriceps, Erector Spinae	4 x 8**

ADVANCED PROGRAM

The Advanced Program is designed only for the elite (male and female) cheerleader. The conditioning requirements for male and female cheerleaders are somewhat different; therefore, we have designed a separate program for each. Both the "non-advanced" male and female cheerleader should start with the beginning program, then move to the intermediate and finally to the advanced program in the time outlined.

The advanced program is difficult, and unless properly executed, injury could result. A Strength Coach should teach you the proper form on the Power Clean, Front Squat and the Weighted Jump Squat. A weight lifting belt should **always** be worn on these exercises as well as on the Push Press and Back Squat. Cheerleaders who train on this Advanced Program should have at least one year of consistent weight training experience on the Intermediate Program, or the equivalent. See page 40 for cycling of sets and reps on the Primary Lifts.

WOMEN'S ADVANCED (ELITE) PROGRAM

Exercise	Figure	Major Muscle Group(s)	Sets x Number of Repetitions
1. Power Clean	4-22	Gluteal Muscles, Quadriceps, Hamstrings, Erector Spinae Gastrocnemius, Trapezius, Deltoids	4 x 8**
2. Bench Press	4-11	Pectorals, Anterior Deltoids, Triceps	4 x 8**
3. Back Squat	4-26	Gluteal Muscles, Quadriceps	4 x 8**
Weighted Jump Squat	4-27	Upper Hamstrings, Erector Spinae, Gastrocnemius	
SUPPLEMENTARY LIFTS:			
4. Close grip Lat Pull-Downs	4-4	Latissimus Dorsi	3 x 8
5. Switch Lunge	4-25	Gluteal Muscles, Quadriceps Upper Hamstrings, Gastrocnemius, Hip Flexors	3 x 8
6. Standing Military Press	4-12	Deltoids, Trapezius, Triceps	3 x 8
7. MB Behind-the-Back	4-13	Deltoids, Trapezius	3 x 8
8. Ab/Adduction	4-17	Hip/Adductors	2 x 10 each
9. Dips	4-9	Triceps, Anterior Deltoids, Pectorals	3 x max.
10. Barbell Curls	4-8	Biceps	3 x 8
11. MB V-Ups	4-1	Hip Flexors/Rectus Abdominis	3 x 8
12. Weighted Back Extensions	4-3	Erector Spinae	3 x 8

MEN'S ADVANCED (ELITE) PROGRAM

Exercise	Figure	Major Muscle Group(s)	Sets x Number of Repetitions
1. Power Clean	4-22	Gluteal Muscles, Quadriceps, Hamstrings, Erector Spinae Gastrocnemius, Trapezius, Deltoids	4 x 8**
2. Bench Press	4-11	Pectorals, Anterior Deltoids, Triceps	4 x 8**
3. Push Press	4-21	Gluteal Muscles, Quadriceps, Upper Hamstrings, Deltoids, Triceps, Gastrocnemius, Trapezius	4 x 8**
SUPPLEMENTARY LIFTS:			
4. Pull Ups	4-4	Latissimus Dorsi	3 x 8
5. Front Squat	4-26	Gluteal Muscles, Quadriceps Upper Hamstrings, Gastrocnemius, Erector Spinae	3 x 8
6. Standing Military Press	4-12	Deltoids	3 x 8
7. MB Behind-the-Back	4-13	Deltoids, Trapezius	3 x 8
8. Barbell Curls	4-8	Biceps	2 x 10 each
9. MB V-Ups	4-1	Hip Flexors, Rectus Abdominis	
10. Seated Deadlift Pull	4-14	Erector Spinae, Gluteal Muscles	3 x max.

PRIMARY LIFTING CYCLES (Sets x Repetitions)

For Intermediate and Advanced Programs

RM = Repetition Maximum

June	(3 weeks)	=	4 x 8	(Approx. 60-65%	1RM)	= Heavy Block
	(1 weeks)	=	4 x 6	(Approx. 60%	1RM)	= Unload Week
July	(3 weeks)	=	4 x 6	(Approx. 70-75%	1RM)	= Heavy Block
	(1 week)	=	4 x 4	(Approx. 70%	1RM)	= Unload Week
Aug.	(3 weeks)	=	4 x 4	(Approx. 80-85%	1RM)	= Heavy Block
	(1 week)	=	4 x 2	(Approx. 80%	1RM)	= Unload Week

Testing

Note: If your Season does not begin the first week in September, continue with this last cycle:

Sept.	(2 weeks)	=	4 x 2	(Approx. 90-95%	1RM)
	(1 week)	=	8-6-4-2	(60-70-80-90%	1RM)

TESTING 1RM = 8-6-3-1-1 (60-70-80-90-100% 1RM)

Before beginning each Primary Exercise with heavy weight, do a light warm up set of 8 repetitions. Then you may begin the 4 x 8 heavy block, setting the weight as heavy as possible while keeping perfect form. The weight should be the same throughout all four sets. Increase the weight (overload) as often as you can throughout the 3 week block, keeping in mind to never sacrifice good lifting form for a heavier weight.

After 3 weeks begin the Unload Week. Basically, this is simply a lighter lifting week. Continue with the same overload; however, only do 4 x 6. The Unload Week is critical in preventing overtraining by allowing the body to recover more fully before the next 3 week block begins.

When it's time to move to the next 3 week heavy block in July, 4 x 6 for 3 weeks, the overload should increase about 10 percent. Continue through the Unload Week which is now 4 x 4 with the same overload.

After you are finished with the 4 x 4 heavy block and the 4 x 2 Unload Week, you may test for a 1 Repetition Maximum (1RM) on the Primary Lifts. Be sure to have spotters assisting, and warm up with an 8-6-3-1 repetition sequence before testing. If your Season doesn't begin early in September, continue the last lifting cycle noted above before testing. After discovering your 1 RM you will be able to set the overload on a percentage (of 1RM) basis during the In-Season Phase. Notice that as the In-Season approaches, intensity (weight) is continually increasing, and volume (repetitions) is simultaneously decreasing.

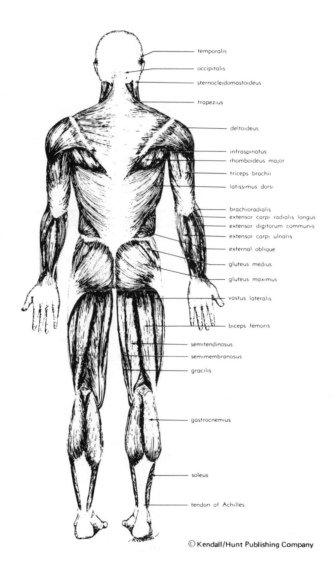

temporalis
occipitalis
sternocleidomastoideus
trapezius
deltoideus
infraspinatus
rhomboideus major
triceps brachii
latissimus dorsi
brachioradialis
extensor carpi radialis longus
extensor digitorum communis
extensor carpi ulnaris
external oblique
gluteus medius
gluteus maximus
vastus lateralis
biceps femoris
semitendinosus
semimembranosus
gracilis
gastrocnemius
soleus
tendon of Achilles

© Kendall/Hunt Publishing Company

STRENGTH AND POWER EXERCISES

HIP FLEXORS/RECTUS ABDOMINIS

V-Ups (Figure 4-1). Lie supine on the floor (Figure 4-1A). Flex at the hips by simultaneously lifting upper and lower body, until you can touch your toes with your hands (Figure 4-1B). Keep legs straight throughout entire exercise. Return to starting position. Only touch floor lightly with hands and feet (do not rest) then start next repetition.

Medicine Ball V-Ups (Not Shown). Same instructions as V-Ups, however, hold a Medicine Ball in your hands. Start with a 4 lb. ball and increase the weight of the ball gradually.

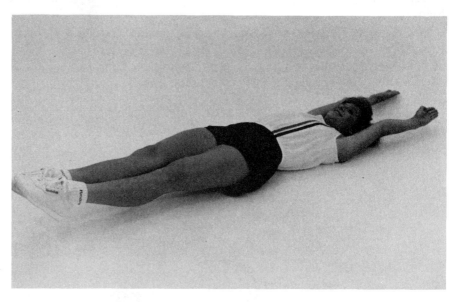

Figure 4-1A

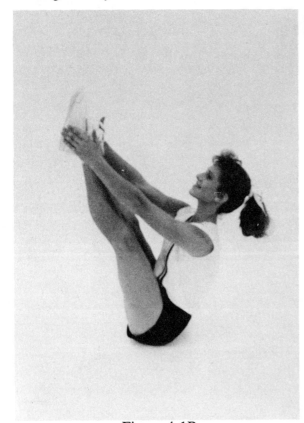

Figure 4-1B

ABDOMINALS AND SIDES

Abdominal Crunch Series

The following four exercises should be done in order. Execute 10 repetitions of each exercise (1 set) before resting. Exercise may be done with feet on the floor, knees bent at a 90% angle or with legs on a bench or chair.

Figure 4-2A. Crunches with a 5 second hold: With lower back in contact with the floor, flex trunk into the "crunch" position (Figure 4-2A) and hold 5 seconds. Return upper back to the floor slowly, and immediately start the next repetition without resting.

Figure 4-2B. Fast Crunches (not shown): Keep lower back in contact with the floor throughout the exercise. This exercise is the same as 5 second hold Crunches, except these are executed quickly, without holding the crunch position at the top.

Figure 4-2C. Twisting Crunches: With the lower back in contact with the floor, flex and twist trunk with opposite elbow to opposite knee (Figure 4-2B). Slowly return upper back to floor. On the next repetition, twist the other direction.

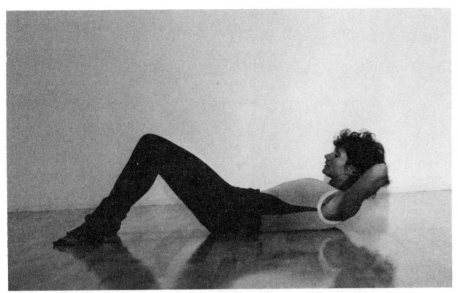

Figure 4-2D. Bent Knee Sit Ups (not shown): With feet fixed on floor, and knees flexed at least 90 degrees, sit all the way up until elbows touch knees at top. Opposite elbow to opposite knee may be touched at the top (twist) as a variation. Return upper back to floor. Start next repetition.

Figure 4-2A

LOWER BACK

Figure 4-3A. Back Extensions on the Floor. Lie face down on the floor, with arms behind your head. Simultaneously lift your head, arms, and chest as well as your feet and legs. Legs should be kept straight. Your back will be in an arched position at the top. Legs should be kept straight. Your back will be in an arched position at the top. Hold this arched position for 2-5 seconds, then slowly (count of four) lower body to the floor. Touch the floor lightly, but do not rest, before moving on to the next repetition.

Figure 4-3B. Back Extensions on Roman Chair. On a Roman chair, place ankles under cross bar. Start with hips flexed at 90 degrees (Figure 4-3B). With a flat back, and hands behind head, extend hips until body is horizontal with the floor (Figure 4-3C). Do NOT arch back at the top. Slowly return to starting position. This should not be a fast jerky exercise, but a slow, controlled movement.

Variation: Weighted Back Extensions. Same instructions as in Back Extensions, however, weight is held either behind the neck or close to the chest. Be sure to start with a very light weight and increase gradually.

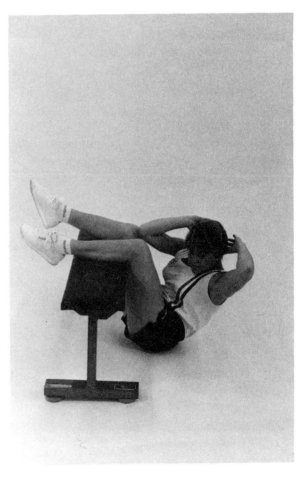

Figure 4-2C

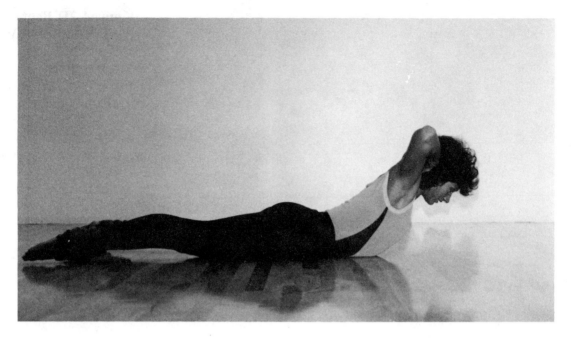

Figure 4-3A

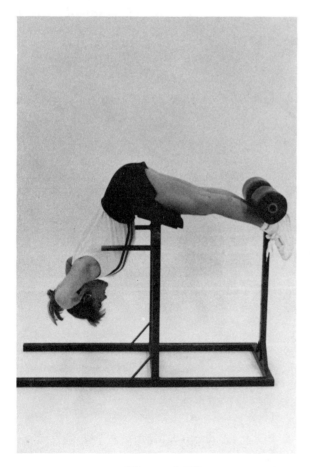

Figure 4-3B

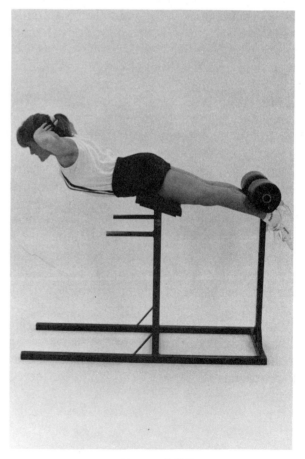

Figure 4-3C

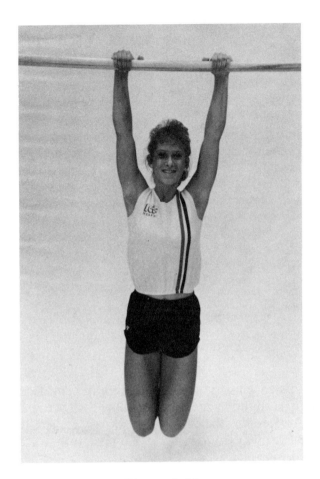

Figure 4-4A

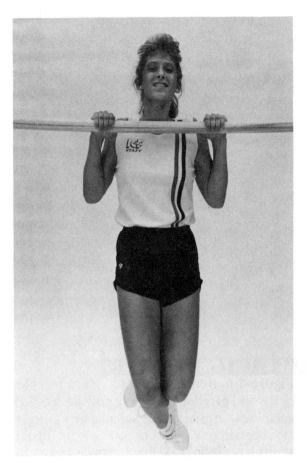

Figure 4-4B

LATISSIMUS DORSI

(The large fan-like muscle which laterally covers most of the back)

Figure 4-4. Pull Ups. Hanging from a bar with an overhand grip about shoulder width apart (Figure 4-4A). Pull body up until chin is over the bar (Figure 4-4B). Slowly let body down until elbows are fully extended.

Figure 4-5. Lat Pull-Down. Sit or kneel under lat bar with an overhand grip greater than shoulder width apart (Figure 4-5A). Pull bar down behind head (Figure 4-5B) and touch base of neck. Slowly let the bar back up until arms are extended once again.

Close Grip Lat Pulldowns (not shown). Sit or kneel under a lat bar using an overhand grip about shoulder width apart (Figure 4-5A). Pull bar down in front of head to collar bone. Slowly let bar back up by extending elbows.

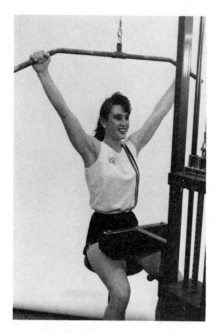

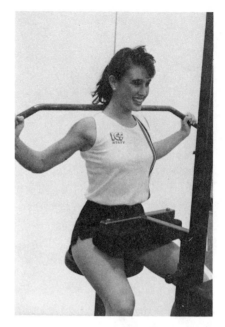

Figure 4-5A   Figure 4-5B

BACK, LATISSIMUS DORSI

Figure 4-6. Bent Over Rows. Place feet shoulder distance apart, with knees slightly bent. Keep back flat and parallel to the floor with your head up. Grip is slightly wider than shoulder distance apart (Bench Press grip would be suitable here) (Figure 4-6A). Keeping the back flat or slightly arched, lift bar to chest (Figure 4-6B). Elbows should lift out to the side away from the body. Slowly return weight to starting position. Breathing: exhale as you lift; inhale as you lower.

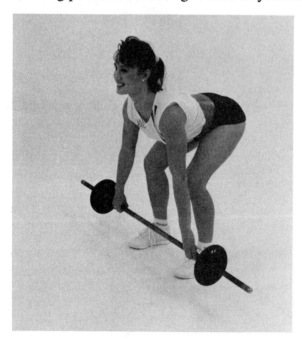

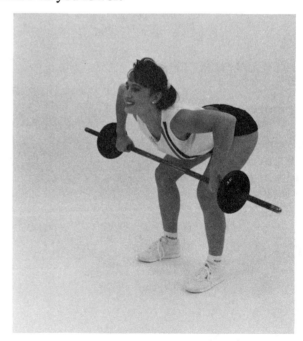

Figure 4-6A   Figure 4-6B

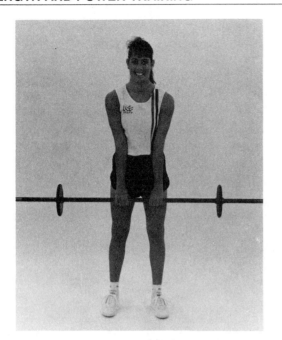
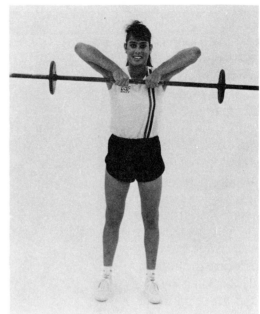

Figure 4-7A   Figure 4-7B

TRICEPS, DELTOIDS, LATISSIMUS DORSI

Figure 4-7. Upright Rows. Standing erect, holding barbell approximately thumbs distance apart with an overhand grip (Figure 4-7A). Leading with the elbows, lift the bar up the torso until it reaches the collar bone (Figure 4-7B). Keep elbows high and to the side. Slowly return to starting position.

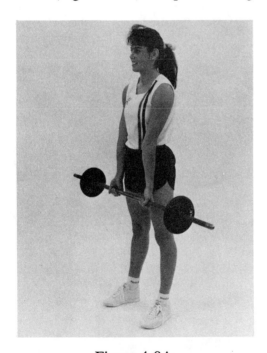
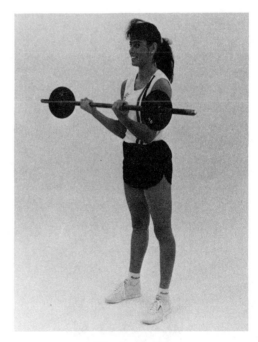

Figure 4-8A   Figure 4-8B

BICEPS

Figure 4-8. Barbell Curl. Hold bar shoulder width apart, palms up (Figure 4-8A). Without moving anything but the elbow joint, lift the bar toward the chest (Figure 4-8B). Do not swing bar or arch back to lift heavier weights. Keep good posture. After bar touches chest slowly lower the bar until arms are extended back into the starting position. Variation: use dumbells in each hand instead of bar.

TRICEPS, ANTERIOR DELTOIDS, PECTORALS

Figure 4-9A Floor Dip
Figure 4-9B. Bench Dips (Not Shown). This is a variation of bar dips. Place hands hip width apart on bench. Support body weight on hands with locked elbows. With legs straight out in front of you, heels on the floor, and hips as close as possible to the bench, lower hips down towards the floor by bending the elbows. After buttocks touch the floor at the bottom, push body back up by extending the arms until you reach the starting position. Breathing: inhale as you lower your body, exhale as you lift it.

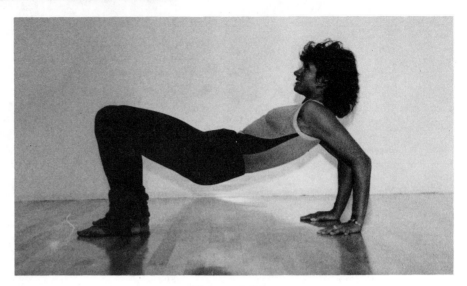

Figure 4-9A

Figure 4-9C, D. Bar Dips. Support body weight on the dip bar to begin the exercise (Figure 4-9C). Slowly lower body toward the floor until chest is in line with the dip bar (Figure 4-9D). Extend arms to lift body back up to the starting position. Breathing: inhale as you lower your body, exhale as you lift it.

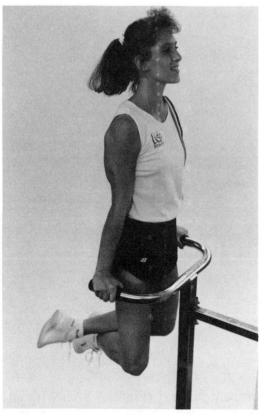

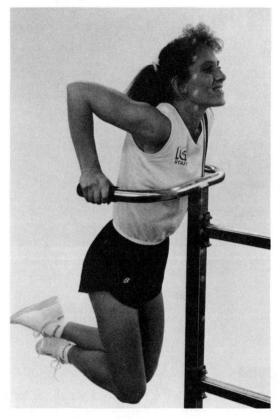

Figure 4-9C   Figure 4-9D

CHEST, DELTOIDS, TRICEPS

Figure 4-10. Push-Ups and Knee Push-Ups. Place hands on the floor slightly wider than shoulder width apart. Lock elbows and support your rigid body (keep abdominal and lower back muscles tight so body is straight) on your hands and the balls of your feet (Figure 4-10A). With elbows bending to the side slowly lower rigid body until chest touches the floor. Elbows should be approximately 90 degrees at the bottom. Push body back up to starting position by extending elbows. Breathing: exhale as you push up, inhale as you lower your body. A beginner's version of the push-up is the knee push up (Figure 4-10B).

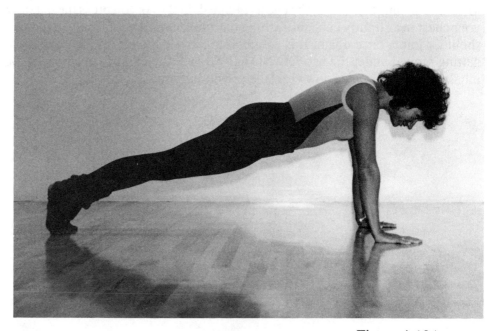

Figure 4-10A

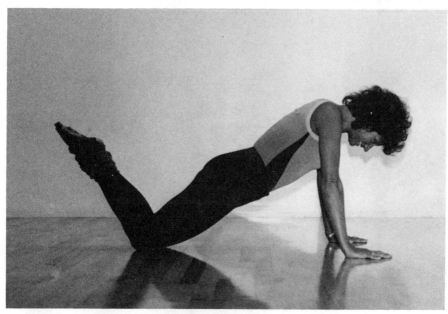

Figure 4-10B

Figure 4-11. Bench Press. Lie down on a flat, horizontal bench, feet flat on the floor with buttocks, upper back and head in contact with the bench throughout the entire exercise. Measure grip width with an empty bar, such that the forearms are perpendicular (i.e. elbow joints at 90 degrees, see Figure 4-11B) to the bar when the bar touches the chest. Start by lifting the bar, or have spotter help "lift off" racks, until it is held directly above the shoulder joints with elbows straight (Figure 4-11A). Slowly lower the bar until it touches the chest (Figure 4-11B). As you press the bar upward it should move from your chest in a slightly concave fashion (curving toward your head) so that it ends up directly over the shoulder joints once again. It is essential to have a spotter on this exercise due to the possibility of getting pinned under the bar. DO NOT BOUNCE the bar off chest, or lift hips off bench. Breathing: inhale as the bar comes down, exhale as you press it.

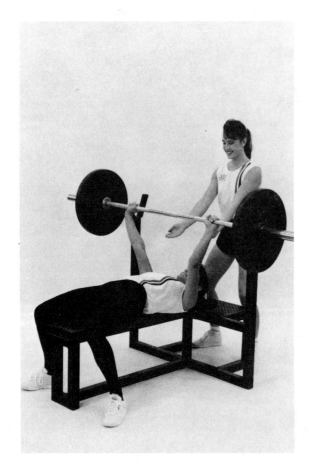

Figure 4-11A

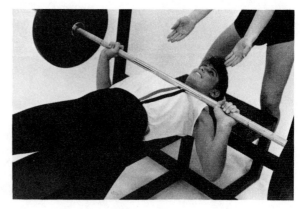

Figure 4-11B

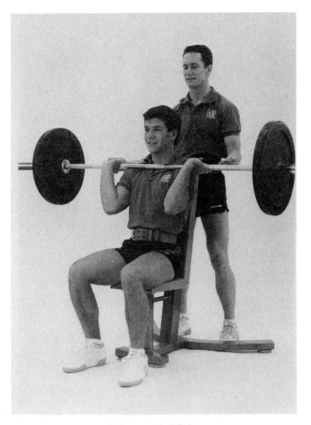

Figure 4-12A

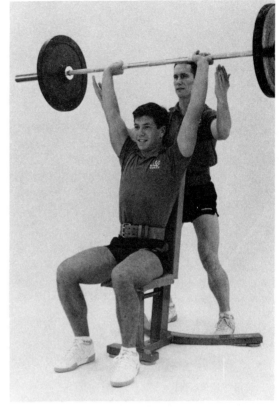

Figure 4-12B

DELTOIDS, TRAPEZIUS, TRICEPS

Figure 4-12. Seated Military Press. Wear a lifting belt on this exercise. Sit on an upright or flat bench. Overhand grip should be slightly wider than shoulder width apart (Figure 4-12A). Keep back flat as you press bar upward over your head (Figure 4-12B). Let bar down slowly to starting position. A spotter is recommended for this exercise.

Figure 4-12C. Standing Military Press. Use the instructions for Seated Military Press. However, this exercise is performed standing erect, feet shoulder width apart. Be sure to keep back flat throughout the entire exercise.

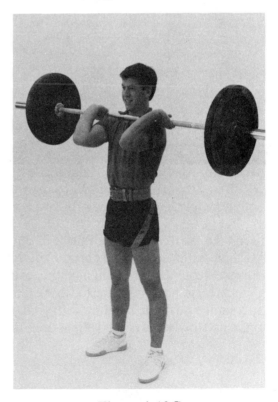

Figure 4-12C

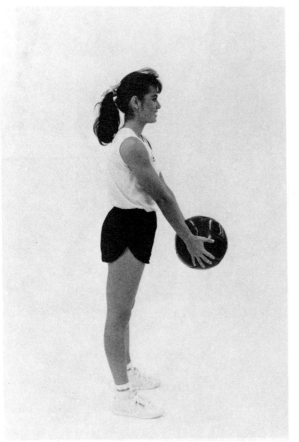

Figure 4-13A

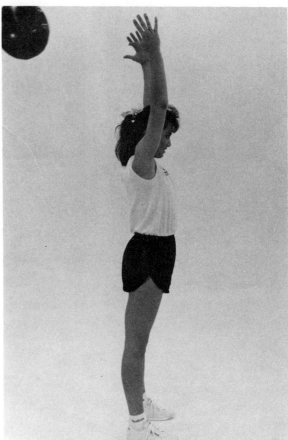

Figure 4-13B

DELTOIDS, TRAPEZIUS

Figure 4-13. Medicine Ball Behind the Back. Stand tall holding ball in front of hips (Figure 4-13A). With straight arms, swing ball up to be thrown overhead backwards to partner (Figure 4-13B). Concentrate on performing a back flip at the end of a tumbling pass.

Figure 4-14. Seated Deadlift Pull (Not Shown). Wear a lifting belt on this exercise. Sit on Seated Row Machine with knees slightly bent. Flex at the hips such that your hands are directly over your feet. The arms are kept straight throughout this entire exercise. Straighten out lower back so that you are sitting erect (torso perpendicular to floor). Continuing with a flat back extend the hips until you are lying in a supine position. Leading with your chest up keep the back flat and return to an erect seated position, then slowly lower the weight until the hands are directly over the feet again.

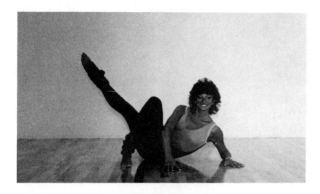

Figure 4-15

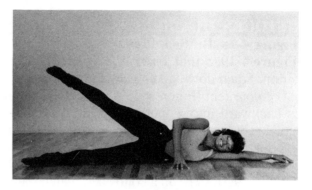

Figure 4-16

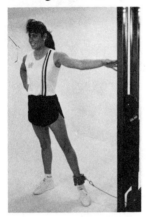

Figure 4-17A

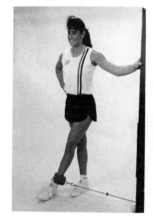

Figure 4-17B

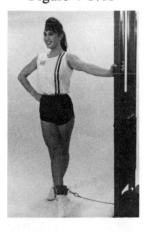

Figure 4-17C

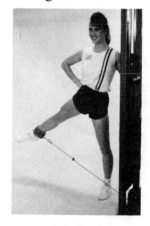

Figure 4-17D

ABDUCTORS, ADDUCTORS

Figure 4-15. Adductor Lift.

Figure 4-16. Abductor Side Leg Raise (Knee Forward).

Figure 4-17. Side Pulls. Abduction: Place ankle strap on outside ankle. With the outside leg starting in a crossed over position in front of the inside leg (Figure 4-17A), abduct or lift leg away from the body to the side, as far as possible (Figure 4-17B). Return leg slowly and cross over in front of the inside leg once again. Switch legs. Adduction: Place ankle strap on inside ankle. Starting with legs about two feet apart (figure 4-17C), adduct or pull inside leg towards outside leg (together) and cross in front as shown in Figure 4-17D. Return slowly to starting position. Switch legs.

BUTTOCKS, QUADRICEPS, HAMSTRINGS

Figure 4-18. Buttock Press.

Figure 4-19. Squat Thrusts. Begin in an erect standing position. Squat down and place your hands on the floor in front of your feet (Figure 4-19A). Quickly extend legs and hips backward into a "push up" position (Figure 4-19B). Recoil knees back up into the squat position (Figure 4-19A). From this deep squat position, jump as high as you can into the air with arms overhead reaching toward the ceiling (Figure 4-19C). Land in a controlled manner and continue directly into the next repetition. Perform this exercise as quickly as possible.

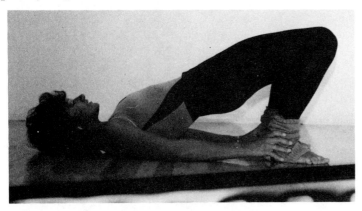

Figure 4-18

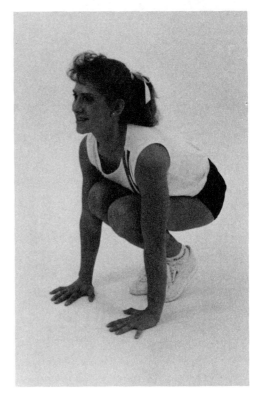

Figure 4-19A

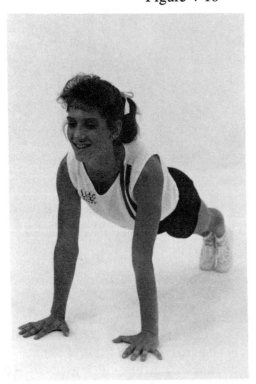

Figure 4-19B

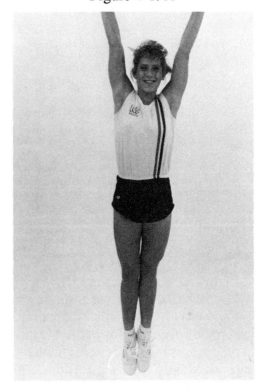

Figure 4-19C

GLUTEUS MAXIMUS

Figure 4-20. High Knee Jump Rope. Jump rope as though you are running (hitting the floor with one foot at a time). Try to lift your knees as high as possible as you "run" (Figure 4-20).

BUTTOCKS, QUADRICEPS, UPPER HAMSTRINGS, CALVES

Figure 4-21. Push Press. Start with the bar resting on the shoulders as in the Power Clean "rack" position (Figure 4-22D). Bend knees slightly (Figure 4-21A), then explode with the legs thrusting the bar upward following through with elbow extension (Figure 4-21B) to final position. Lower bar back to the starting position in a controlled manner.

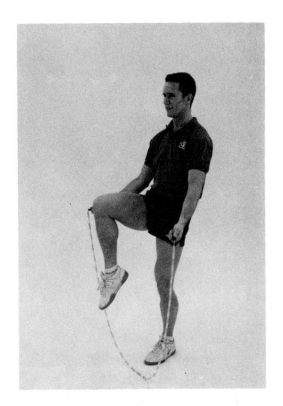

Figure 4-20

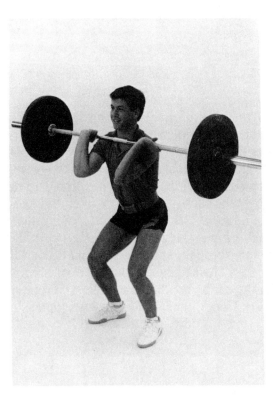

Figure 4-21A

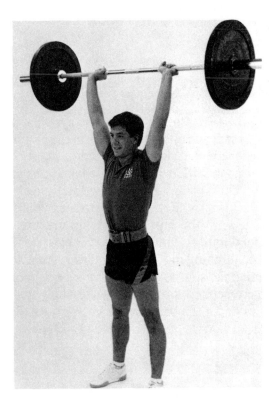

Figure 4-21B

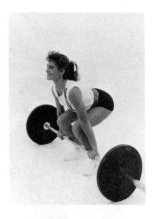

Figure 4-22A

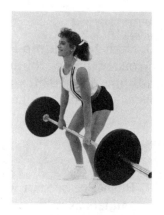

Figure 4-22B

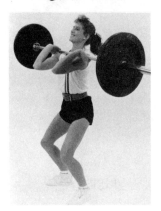

Figure 4-22C

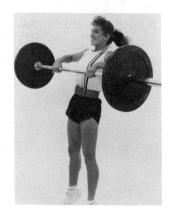

Figure 4-22D

BUTTOCKS, QUADRICEPS, HAMSTRINGS, ERECTOR SPINAE

Figure 4-22. Power Clean. Always wear a lifting belt on this exercise. If at all possible use bumper plates (made of rubber) as shown in the picture. Place feet shoulder distance apart, with weight on the balls of the feet. Grip should be comfortably outside legs slightly wider than shoulder width apart. Be sure your shoulders are over the bar at this point. Shins should be touching bar, back flat or slightly arched, chest up and eyes focused straight ahead (Figure 4-22A) for the starting position. Lift the bar over the knees while continuing to keep your shoulders over the bar. After the bar is over the knee caps, explode with the hips (bring them towards the bar) (Figure 4-22B and 4-22C) keeping the arms extended until full hip extension is reached. This explosive hip and leg extension is very similar to a vertical jumping motion. After the hips reach full extension, shrug the shoulders up and lift the elbows up and to the side so the bar travels straight up the body very close to the torso (Figure 4-22C). When the bar reaches approximately chest height move under the bar by bending the knees and rotating the elbows under the bar in a "rack" position (Figure 4-22D). Uncoil the bar the same way it was lifted.

QUADRICEPS, HAMSTRINGS
Figure 4-23. Side Kicks.

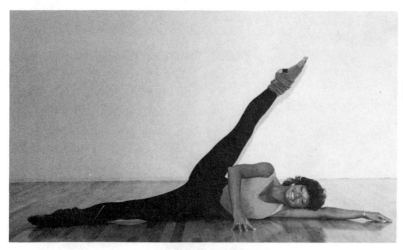

Figure 4-23

QUADRICEPS
Figure 4-24. Leg Extension. From a seated position (Figure 4-24A) extend legs in a controlled manner (count of two) with ankles flexed (Figure 4-24B). After full knee extension is reached, slowly (count of four) flex the knees back to the starting position.

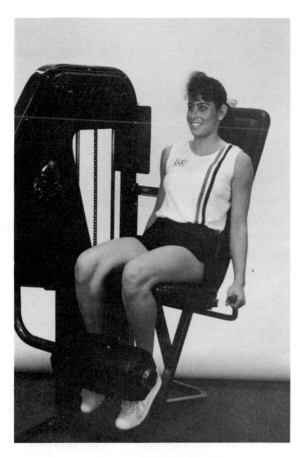

Figure 4-24A

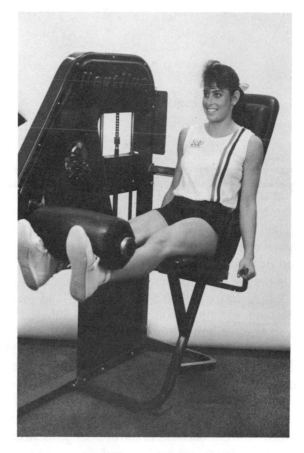

Figure 4-24B

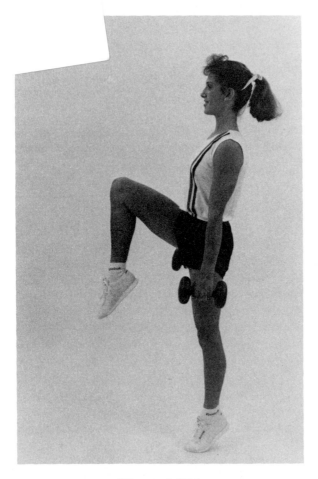 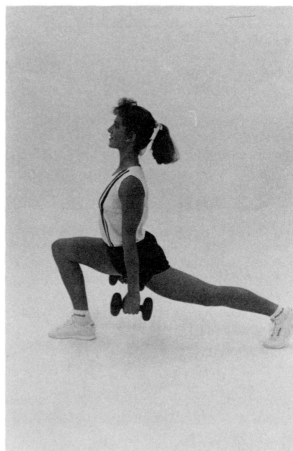

Figure 4-25A   Figure 4-25B

QUADRICEPS, HAMSTRINGS, BUTTOCKS

Figure 4-25. Lunges (Walking). After several workouts using only body weight, this exercise can be done with dumbbells (as shown) or with a barbell behind the neck on the shoulders. From the starting position (Figure 4-25A) take a large step forward so that the knee is directly over the toes (Figure 4-25B). Keep head and chest up throughout the entire movement. Back leg may bend slightly depending upon flexibility, however, try to keep it as straight as possible. Push up and back off of front leg and bring the back leg forward driving the knee up quickly and fully extend hip at the top. Releve (go up on ball of foot) with the opposite leg, and prepare for the next step. Go down slow and up fast. Breathing: exhale as you step forward, inhale as you return to the standing position (Figure 4-25B). This is an excellent exercise to do: (1) up a ramp or hill if weights are not available, or (2) as a variation.

Figure 4-25C. Variation: Split Lunges (Not Shown). Be sure you are warmed up and stretched out before attempting this exercise. This exercise should be done without weight. Begin in the deep lunge position (Figure 4-25B) with hands on the hips or comfortably hanging at your side. Keeping your chest up and eyes focused straight ahead, explode with both legs simultaneously, jumping up as high as possible. Switch legs quickly in mid air so that you can land in a deep lunge position with the other leg forward. Elite cheerleaders can challenge themselves further by doing a Double Split lunge, where the legs switch front and back in mid air, similar to a switch leap in gymnastics.

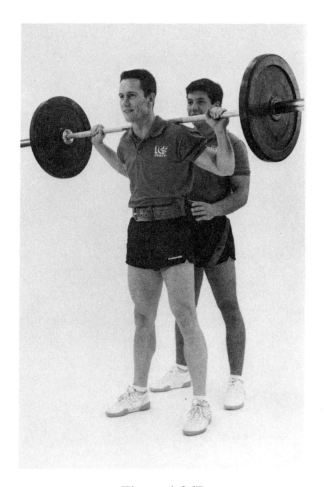

Figure 4-26B

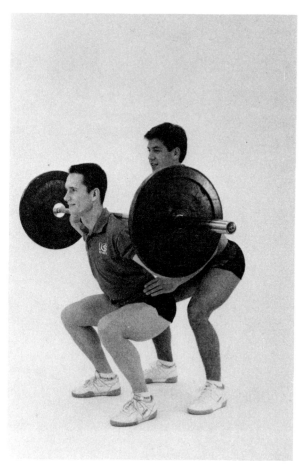

Figure 4-26C

QUADRICEPS, HAMSTRINGS

Figure 4-26A. Free Hand Squat (Not Shown). Same instructions as Back Squat, however, no weight is used. Place hands on hips or cross in front of chest for better balance. Breathing: inhale as you go down, exhale as you go up.

Figure 4-26B,C. Back Squat. Place feet slightly wider than shoulder width, toes pointed slightly out (Figure 4-26B). With back flat or slightly arched, eyes focused straight ahead, and chest up, squat until thighs are parallel with the floor (Figure 4-26C). Be sure to keep back tight, and heels on the floor. Avoid leaning forward, in fact, keep your weight towards your heels. As you watch yourself in the mirror be sure that your knees are going directly over your toes. Rise from the squat position by pushing hips forward, keeping back tight and chest up. Extend hips fully at the top by squeezing the buttocks before beginning next repetition. After you have perfect form and balance, go through releve (up on the balls of the feet) at the end of each repetition. Lower to a flat footed stance before starting the next repetition. Concentrate on going down slow and coming up fast.

Figure 4-26D. Front Squat. Same instructions as Back Squat, however, the bar is held in front of the shoulders in a Power Clean "rack" position (Figure 4-22D).

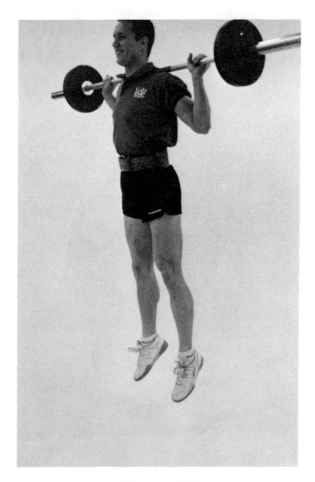

Figure 4-27A

Figure 4-27. Jump Squat. Same instructions throughout the lowering phase of the Back Squat. Once the parallel position is reached at the bottom, explode with the legs and jump as high as possible (Figure 4-27A) keeping back tight and chest up. Fully extend hips at the top by squeezing the buttocks. Landing should be controlled.

Figure 4-27B. Free Hand Jump Squat (Not Shown). Same instructions as Jump Squat, however, no weight is used. Hands can be on hips, or cross arms in front of chest.

HAMSTRINGS

Figure 4-28. Back Kicks.

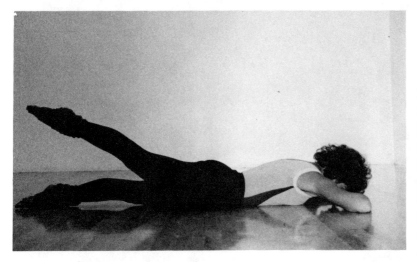

Figure 4-28

Figure 4-29. Leg Curl. Lie on bench with knee caps slightly beyond pad (Figure 4-29A), and head up. Bring heels toward buttocks in a controlled manner (count of two). From the fully flexed position of the knees (Figure 4-29B) slowly (count of four) let the cross bar down until legs are extended.

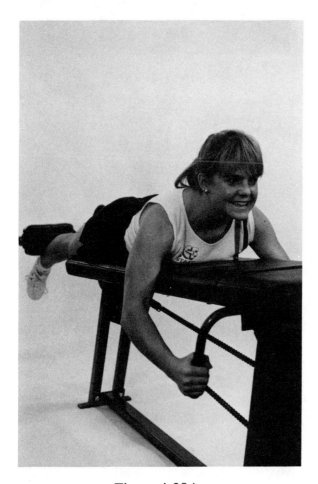

Figure 4-29A

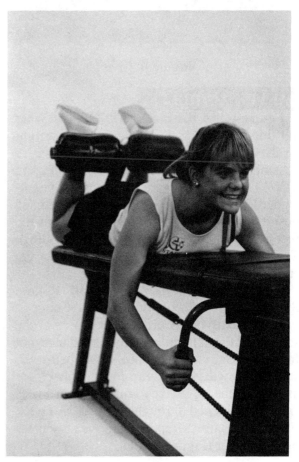

Figure 4-29B

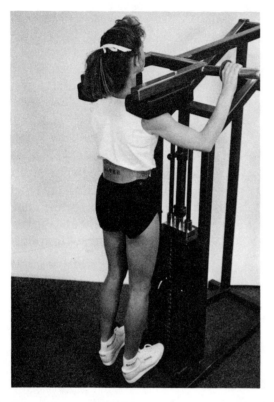

Figure 4-30A

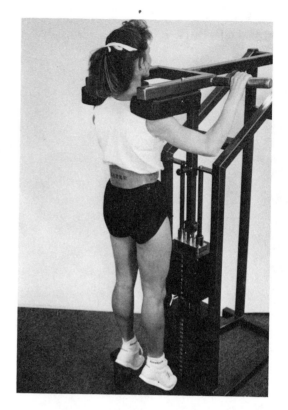

Figure 4-30B

CALVES, ACHILLES

Figure 4-30A,B. Machine Calf Raises. Wear a lifting belt during this exercise. With weight on the balls of the feet, lower heels as far as possible into a calf "stretched" position (Figure 4-30A). Be sure knees are not locked (hyperextended) in this exercise. After the stretched position is reached, rise up on the balls of the feet (releve) as high as possible (Figure 4-30B). Then slowly begin to lower heels into the stretched position.

Figure 4-30C. Floor/Stair Calf Raises. Stand with the balls of your feet on the edge of a step so that your heels are hanging over the step. Hold the handrail slightly for balance, not for a push. Start with your heels as far below the step as they will go. Press up until your heels are as high in the air as they will go. Your knees should be locked throughout. VARIATION: Floor Calf Raises. Repeat as above only press up from floor (Figure 4-30C).

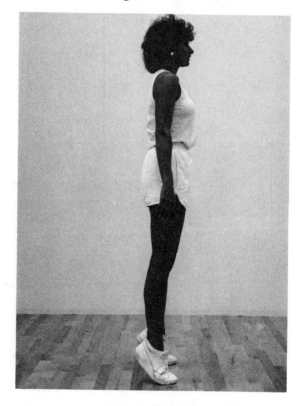

Figure 4-30C

FLEXIBILITY
Chapter Five

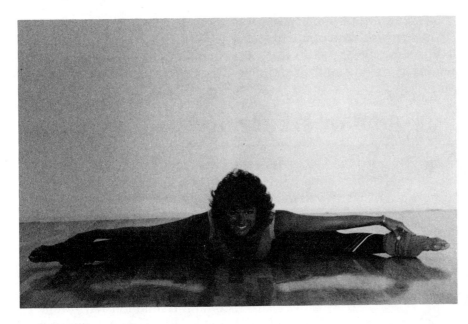

Flexibility is a key component of fitness that, in addition to endurance and strength and power, greatly affects your skill development and overall cheering ability. Correct stretching before practice and performance will decrease your chance of injury as well as increase your overall physical skills. Better yet, you can develop excellent flexibility through simple daily stretching and, as long as you are committed, you'll soon see great results! Let's learn the basic principles of flexibility, set our game plan and get started!

> *"We always stretch out a little before practicing jumps and gymnastics, but does stretching affect any specific skill area?"*

FLEXIBILITY AND PERFORMANCE

Flexibility involves the length of a muscle from its origin to its insertion. The longer a muscle is from origin to insertion, the more fluent and productive the range of motion will be. Proper stretching increases flexibility; muscles are lengthened and muscular tension is reduced, thereby allowing free movement of your joints. And, as adequate flexibility increases the range of motion of various parts of your body, it decreases the muscular effort necessary for performing many cheering skills. Remember, the greater your range of motion, the greater your ability to perform many cheering skills.

If you are serious about performing at your best, you need to develop muscular competence. We cannot stress enough that properly stretching your muscles is a key factor in the success of your conditioning workouts. Your level of flexibility also directly affects your ability to perform specific cheering skills such as heel stretches, kicks, lunges, jumps, stunts and gymnastics.

> *"I am concerned about preventing injuries on my squad. Do flexibility stretches cut down on the possibility of injuries?"*

INJURY PREVENTION

Stretching can help prevent musculoskeletal injuries. These injuries are often caused by poor flexibility and are all too often a result of inadequate stretching before attempting skills. Although we see a great number of problems from inadequate stretching, injuries can also be caused by too much stretching. Muscles are easily strained! Make sure your squad incorporates correct stretching technique in all your practices and performances. The following safety tips may be helpful reminders to you and your squad.

1. Your chance of injury increases **without** proper stretching.
2. Your chance of injury increases **with improper** stretching.
3. Applying **too much force** to a muscle or joint is improper stretching.
4. **Pain indicates too much force** is being applied and should never be a part of stretching (this includes partner stretching).

METHODS OF STRETCHING

"Everybody on our squad stretches before practice, but we all do different things and we don't know exactly what we are stretching. Do different types of stretching make a difference?"

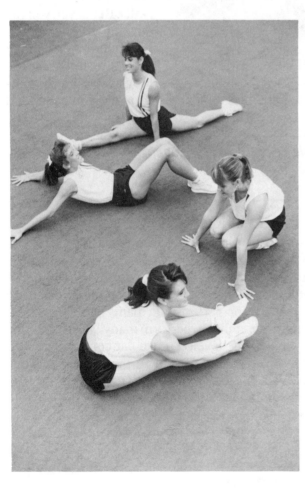

STATIC STRETCHING

Several stages of stretching are important to understand. Static stretching is when a muscle is slowly stretched until a mild tension is felt. This should be held for 10-30 seconds. Tension should subside as you hold the position. If the tension results in pain, ease off slightly until the tension level is comfortable. This stage reduces muscular tightness and prepares your muscles group for the developmental stage of stretching.

DEVELOPMENTAL STRETCHING

Tension in the muscle group should be increased slightly in the developmental stage of stretching. This is similar to the static stretch; however, here you are increasing the effort put on your muscles. This tension should also be held for 10-30 seconds.

Make sure both stages of stretching are executed slowly. The slow tension or movement recruits a higher number of muscle fibers. Keep your **breathing** as normal as possible in both stages. Exhale while you apply tension and inhale as the stretch is about to occur. Never hold your breath while stretching as this may cause a slight increase in blood pressure.

HYPER OR FORCED STRETCHING

The most productive as well as potentially dangerous stretching is hyper (forced). In this type of stretch, the overload principle is involved. This means your muscle is asked to bear more tension through carefully applied force than is normally required. PNF techniques (explanation follows) are ideal in this form of stretching.

PNF (proprioceptive neuromuscular facilitation) is a technique used by physiatrists for therapeutic exercise and can be applied as a method of forced stretching in cheerleading. The three step PNF method of forced stretching is basically **contract-relax-contract.** More specifically:

1. Note the body part to be stretched and apply light force by partner for ten seconds. (Contract)
2. Relax the muscle without any force applied by partner, then stretch the muscle immediately. (Relax)
3. Apply light force to muscle again. (Contract)

WHEN AND WHAT TO STRETCH
GENERAL CONDITIONING AND CASUAL STRETCHING

Your overall conditioning workout should include flexibility exercises along with your endurance, power, and strength training. These flexibility exercises should be done consistently even if no games or practices are scheduled, and even if you are not working on endurance or strength! In fact, casual stretching can be done on a daily basis in a variety of environments: while you are watching T.V., studying, reading or during your free time at home or school. Along with helping to develop your overall fitness level, stretching relieves tension and stress. So the next time you're preparing for a big test, stretch!

> *"Every time I do high kicks or knee lunges in our pom routines, my legs are always stiff. Any advice?"*

PRACTICES, PERFORMANCES AND APPLIED STRETCHING

One of the most common mistakes made by athletes is beginning strenuous activity without first warming up and stretching out their muscles. Without a doubt cheerleading physical skills are strenuous, so there is no excuse for omitting this important step! Decrease your chance of injury each time you cheer by reminding yourself to "stretch first."

Although flexibility exercises should be included in your general workouts, stretching before practices and performances should be mandatory. Often referred to as applied stretching, this will take more time and effort than the casual stretching used in your overall conditioning program. Sometimes you ,may need to spend extra time warming up a particular area of the body that you plan to workout harder than usual. For example, if you will be working on heel stretches during practice, spend extra time warming up your legs. Or, during a game when you are about to perform a tumbling pass, take time for a quick stretch of your wrists, neck, and ankles. Always get a complete warm-up before you begin practice or a performance.

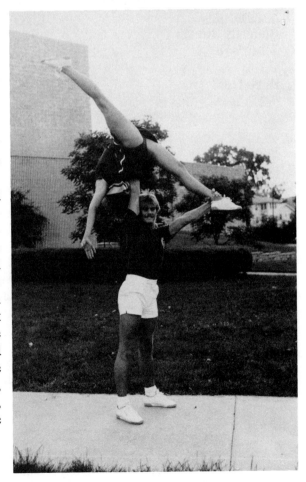

STRETCHING PROGRESSION

Although stretching programs vary, many sports medicine experts agree and recommend that body parts should be stretched in a specific order for the best results. It is recommended that you **begin with the large muscle groups and finish with the smaller groups.** Keeping the blood flow in the target area is important and will be accomplished if you follow the principle of large to small muscle groups listed below. A simple way to remember the order of stretching is to start at the feet and work your way up. Stretch one area thoroughly before moving on to another.

A. LOWER BODY
   1. Hip Flexors
   2. Quadriceps
   3. Hamstrings
   4. Ankles
   5. Achiles

B. UPPER BODY
   1. Back
   2. Chest
   3. Shoulders
   4. Neck
   5. Triceps
   6. Biceps
   7. Wrists

LOWER BODY
FLEXIBILITY EXERCISES

HIP FLEXORS (Gluteus maximus - buttocks)

Beginning	Intermediate	Advanced
Butterfly Stretch 5-1a, 5-1b	Squat Stretch 5-3a, 5-3b	Lunge Stretch 5-5a, 5-5b
Knee Hold 5-2	Runner's Stretch 5-4	Triangle Sit 5-6

HAMSTRINGS

Beginning	Intermediate	Advanced
Leg Raise 5-7	Straddle Side 5-9	Side Splits 5-11
Straddle Stretch Front 5-8a, 5-8b, 5-8c	Pike 5-10	Straddle Splits 5-12

QUADRICEPS

Beginning	Intermediate	Advanced
Quad Pull Back 5-13	Double Pull Back 5-14	Advanced Quad Knee Lunge 5-16
	Partner Pull Back Extension 5-15a, 5-15b	Quad Knee Tuck 5-17

CALVES (Gastrocnemius)

Beginning	Intermediate	Advanced
Partner Step	Floor Step	Hold Floor Step
5-18	5-19	5-19 (not shown)
		60 seconds

ANKLE, PLANTAR FLEXOR

Beginning	Intermediate	Advanced
Ankle Rolls	Partner Lean	Single Lean
5-20	5-21	5-22
	Plantar Stretch	
	5-23	

UPPER BODY
BACK

Beginning	Intermediate	Advanced
Bridge Up	Torso Twist	Lat Pull
5-24a, 5-24b	5-25	5-26

SIDES

Beginning	Intermediate	Advanced
Side Pull	Straddle Reach	
5-27	5-28	

CHEST

Beginning	Intermediate	Advanced
Chest Press	Hyper Chest	Airplane
5-29	5-30a, 5-30b	5-31

SHOULDERS

Beginning	Intermediate	Advanced
Arm Circles	Wish Bone	Hyper Shoulder
5-32	5-34	5-35
Waist Pull		Bottom Slide
5-33a, 5-33b		5-36

ARMS

Beginning	Intermediate	Advanced
Wrist Rolls	Wrist Press	
5-37	Palm Down Left, Palm Down Right	
	5-38	

NECK

Beginning	Intermediate	Advanced
	Neck Stretch	
	5-39	

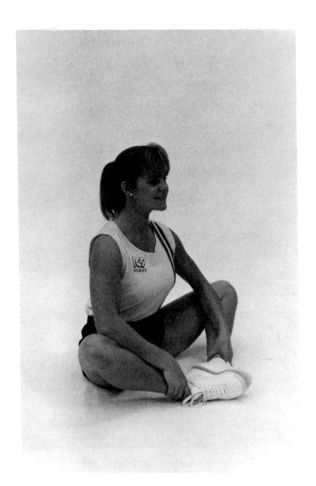

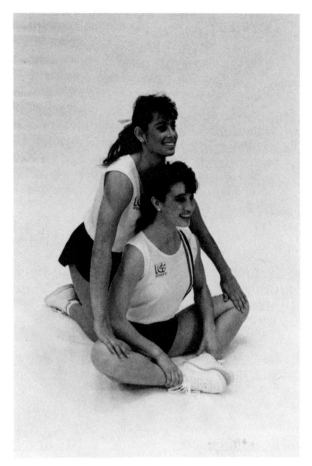

Figure 5-1a   Figure 5-1b

Figure 5-1a, 5-1b. BUTTERFLY STRETCH. Start in a sitting position with soles of feet together, knees turned out; head up; shoulders back. Hands pull ankles back slightly then gently press elbows down on knee (5-1a). **Variation: Partner Stretch**—start in the same position as in the single Butterfly Stretch (5-1a). Partner assists in pressing the knees while slightly pressing forward on back (5-1b), hold for the stretch.

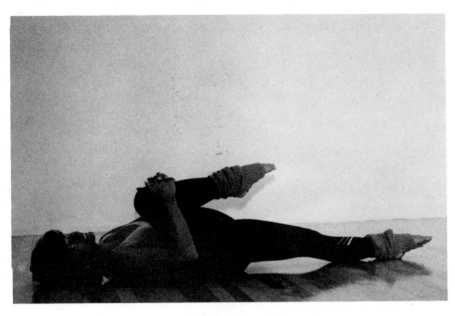

Figure 5-2

Figure 5-2. KNEE HOLD. Start in supine position (on back), bend one knee to chest and extend opposite leg. Grasp hands over knee and pull gently towards head, hold for the stretch. Repeat on opposite leg.

Figure 5-3a, 5-3b. SQUAT STRETCH. Start in squat position with feet double shoulder width apart; knees and feet turned out, back straight, head up (5-3a) hands on knees. Drop bottom towards floor, head must remain up and shoulders back, hold for the stretch. Hands reach in toward heels.

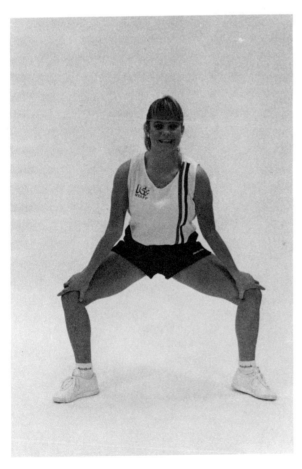

Figure 5-3a

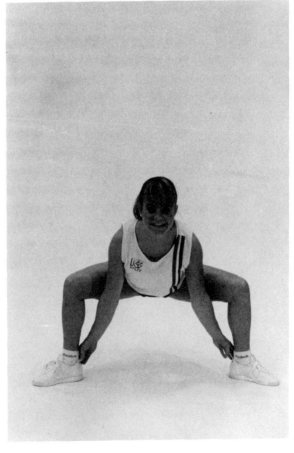

Figure 5-3b

Figure 5-4. RUNNER STRETCH. Starting position: Start in deep lunge position, foot in front of bent knee, back leg straight, head and shoulders up and hands support on floor. Action: Gently press hip slightly towards floor and hold for the stretch.

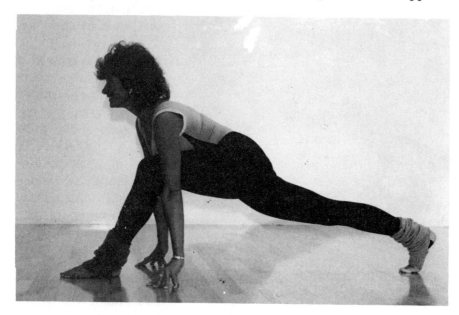

Figure 5-5a, 5-5b. KNEE LUNGE STRETCH. Starting position: Knee lunge position (5-5a), foot in front of bent knee, head up and shoulders back. Action: (5-5b) Press hips toward floor, hold for the stretch.

Figure 5-4

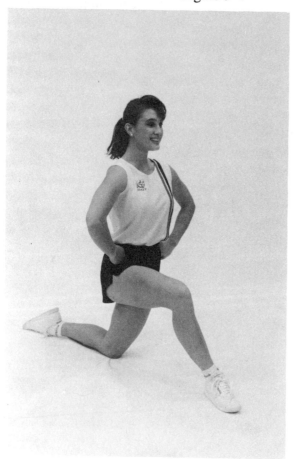

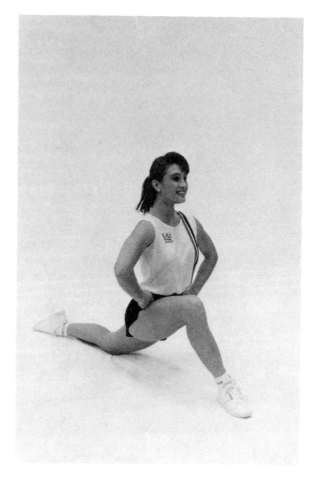

Figure 5-5a

Figure 5-5b

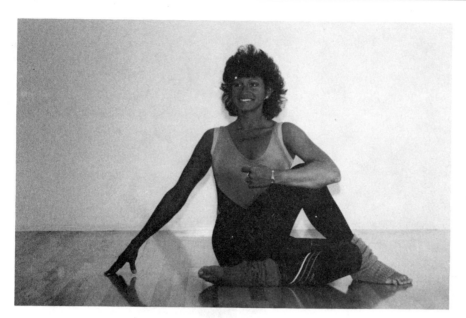

Figure 5-6

Figure 5-6. TRI-ANGLE SIT. Starting position: Sit on floor, bend left knee and pull left foot towards bottom. Cross right foot over left knee, shoulders back, head up, hook left arm around right knee and balance with right hand. Action: Pull knee towards body and hold for the stretch.

Figure 5-7. LEG RAISE. Lie flat on back, extend one leg straight on floor, grasp opposite leg with both hands, keep leg straight (5-7). Pull straight leg gently to chest and hold for the stretch.

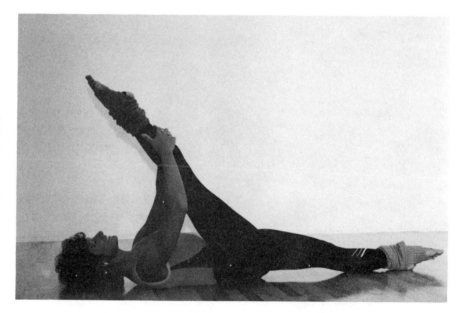

Figure 5-7

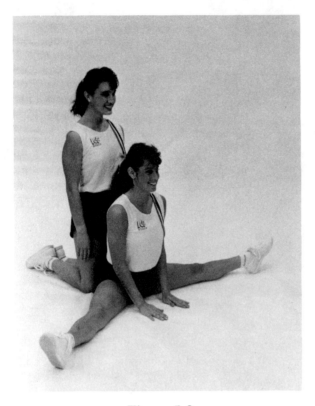

Figure 5-8a

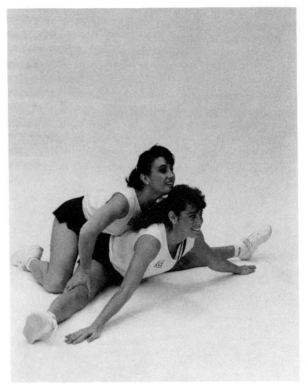

Figure 5-8b

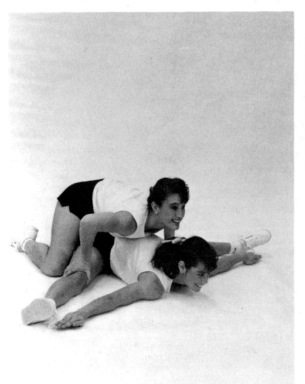

Figure 5-8c

Figure 5-8a,b,c. STRADDLE STRETCH FRONT. Sit on floor with legs in straddle position, toes pointed, knees up. Partner on knees behind (5-8a). Reach hands toward feet, head up, press toward floor (5-8b). Partner keeps hands on knees to stabilize knees in vertical position (don't allow knees to roll forward). (5-9c) Continue stretch to floor with partner pushing on lower back while stabilizing the knees. Hold for the stretch.

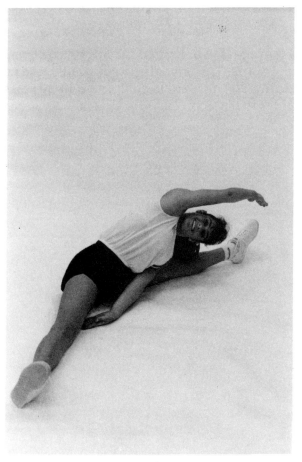

Figure 5-9

Figure 5-9. STRADDLE SIDE. Sit on floor, legs in straddle position, toes pointed, knees up. Reach arm up and over toward opposite foot with chest remaining open. Hold for the stretch.

Figure 5-10. PIKE. Sit on floor, legs together, knees slightly bent and turned out (to avoid lower back stress). Stretch hands forward, chin up, flat back. At maximum point of stretch, relax upper body by curving back and dropping head. Hold for the stretch (5-10).

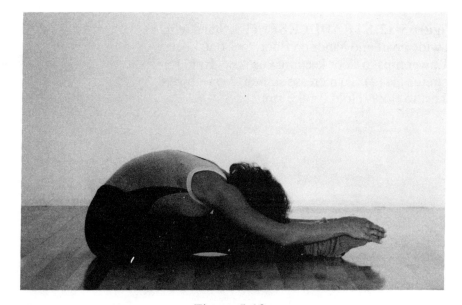

Figure 5-10

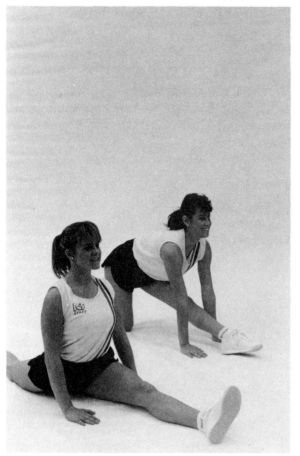

Figure 5-11

Figure 5-11. SIDE SPLITS. Start on knees and straighten one leg forward between hands, head up. Slide front leg forward to complete split by pressing hips to the floor. Hold for stretch.

Figure 5-12. STRADDLE SPLITS. Stand with legs wide apart and hands on floor, toes out, knees up. Lower hips to floor keeping knees up. Hold for the stretch (5-12). To increase stretch, drop elbows or chest to floor. Hold for the stretch.

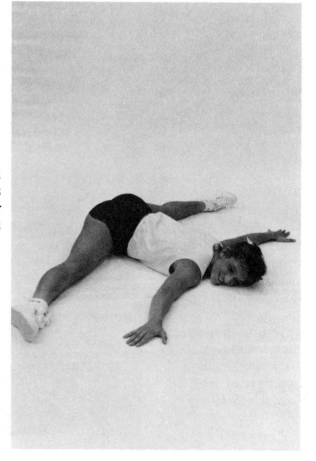

Figure 5-12

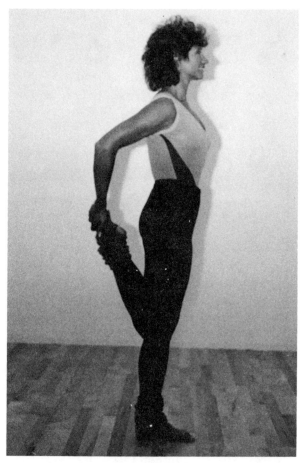

Figure 5-13. QUAD PULL BACK. Stand on left leg, bend right leg back and grasp foot with right hand. Gently pull foot up and back. Hold for the stretch.

Figure 5-13

Figure 5-14. DOUBLE PULL BACK. Lie on stomach and bend both knees back, grasp feet with hands keeping head up (5-14). Pull feet up and toward back and hold for the stretch.

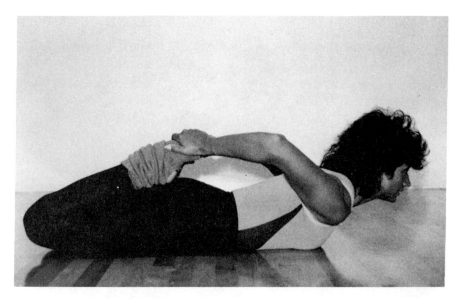

Figure 5-14

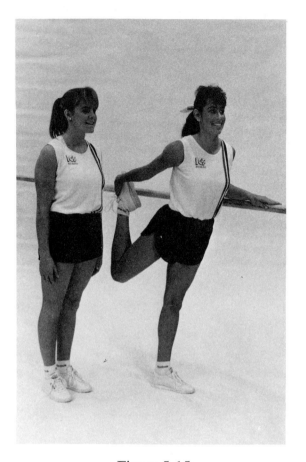

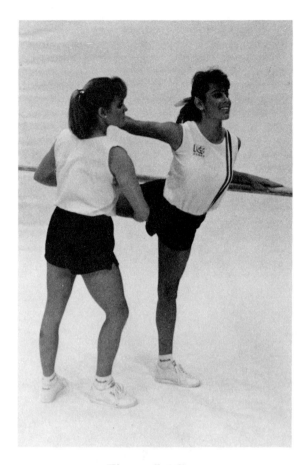

Figure 5-15a   Figure 5-15b

Figure 5-15a, 5-15b. Using chair, bar, or wall for balance, stand on foot closest to wall and lift opposite leg while grabbing foot with same side hand (5-15a). Lift foot up and back. Partner assists by hooking one arm under upper thigh and the other hand above the knee and lift (5-15b).

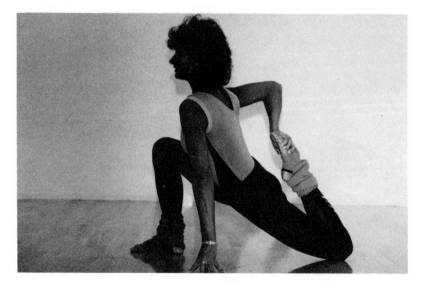

Figure 5-16. AD-VANCED QUAD KNEE. Start in a deep knee lunge with foot in front of knee. Gently shift weight forward so that contact to the floor is above the knee. Grasp foot and pull toward lower back using opposite arm for balance, head up, shoulders back. Hold for the stretch.

Figure 5-16

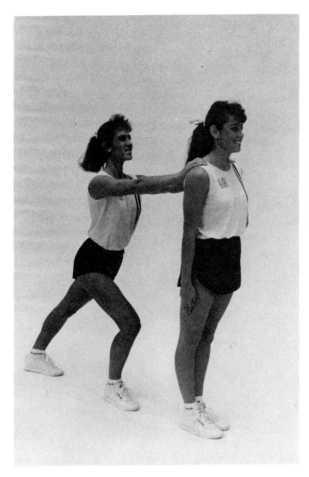

Figure 5-18

Figure 5-18. PARTNER STEP. Using partner for balance, begin in deep lunge position, head up, shoulders back, feet flat on floor (5-18). Lower hips toward floor keeping back leg straight, heel down. Hold for the stretch.

Figure 5-19. FLOOR STEP. Start on hands and feet with feet together. Bend one leg with weight on straight leg. Press heel of straight leg to floor. Hold for the stretch.

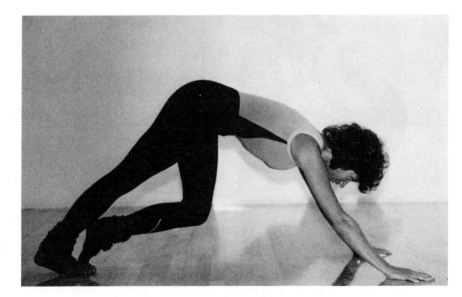

Figure 5-19

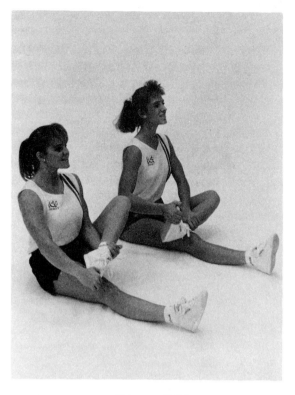

Figure 5-20

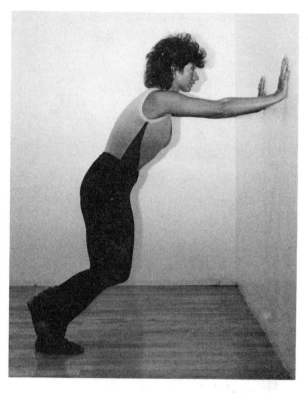

Figure 5-21

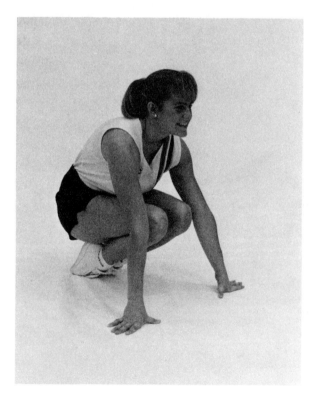

Figure 5-22

Figure 5-20. ANKLE ROLLS. Sit on floor with one leg straight, opposite knee turned out with foot close to body. Grasp under ankle with one hand and grasp toes with opposite hand. Slowly circle foot several times with hand assisting so maximum range of motion can be completed.

Figure 5-21. PARTNER LEAN. Using partner or wall for balance, knee forward on one leg with kne bent; hook opposite foot behind ankle. Bend knee forward pressing heel down. Hold for the stretch.

Figure 5-22. PLANTAR STRETCH (TOE POINT). Start on hands and knees with feet and hands together, toes pointed behind. Lean back, dropping bottom towards toes and lifting knees. Hold for the stretch.

Figure 5-23. SINGLE LEAN. Start with hands and feet on floor, feet together. Hook one foot behind opposite ankle; slowly bend knee. Hold for the stretch.

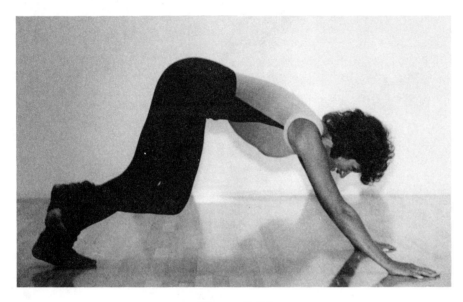

Figure 5-23

Figure 5-24a,b. BRIDGE UP. Start flat on back, knees bent, feet close to body, hands on floor close to head, elbows up. Press upward straightening arms (5-24a) and lifting hips. (5-24b) Straighten both legs pushing shoulders over hands while partner assists by pulling and lifting the waist. Hold for the stretch.

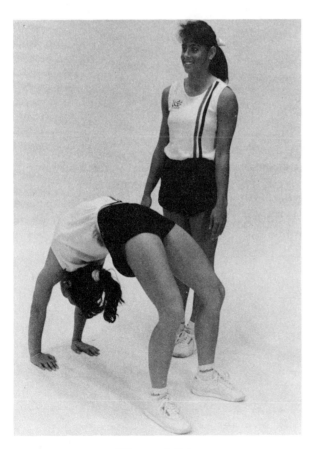

Figure 5-24a

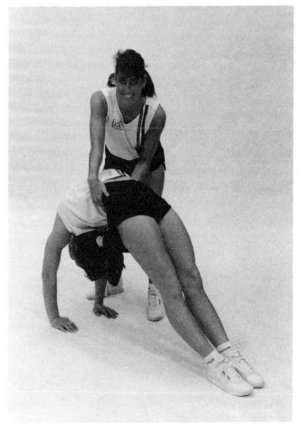

Figure 5-24b

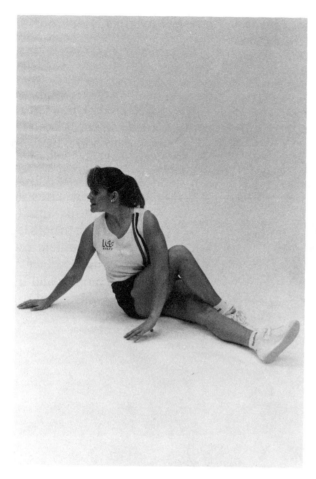

Figure 5-25

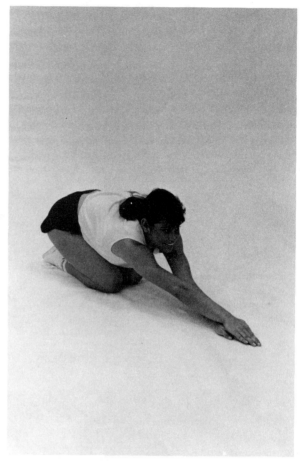

Figure 5-26

Figure 5-25. TORSO TWIST. Sit on floor with one leg straight and opposite leg bent—crossed over knee with foot flat on floor. (5-25) Cross opposite arm over bent leg. Twist upper body in same direction, balance with opposite arm, hold for the stretch. Repeat on opposite side.

Figure 5-26. CAT PULL. Start on floor on hands and knees; hips directly over knees; arms stretched out in front of body with one hand on top of the other. Shift weight backward and sit. Simultaneously while sitting, pull bottom hand back from top hand and top hand pressing down to hold bottom hand (do not lose contact). Hold for the stretch. Repeat opposite side.

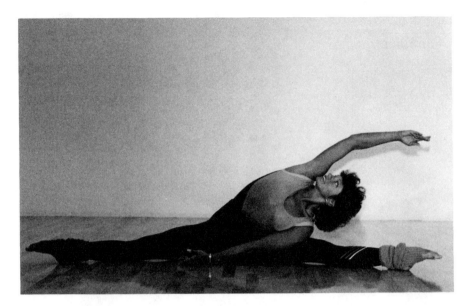

Figure 5-28

Figure 5-28. STRADDLE REACH. Same description as 5-9.

Figure 5-29. CHEST PRESS. Lie face down on floor in push-up position, hands close to chest. Press hips to floor while straightening arms, back arches, head up. Hold for the stretch.

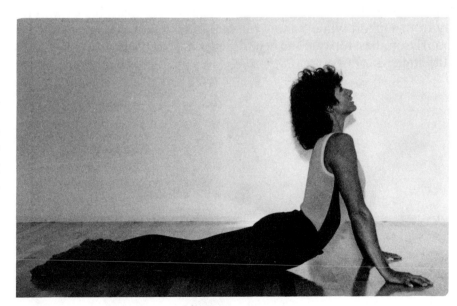

Figure 5-29

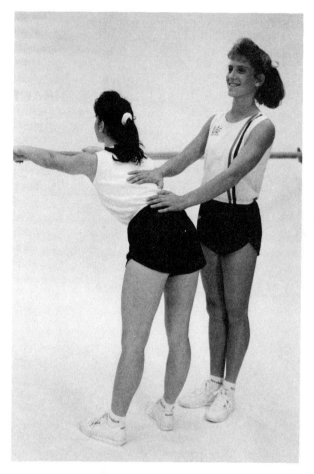

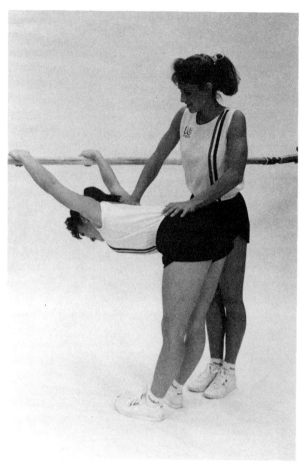

Figure 5-30a   Figure 5-30b

Figure 5-30a,b. HYPER CHEST. (5-30a) Using chair, bar or wall for balance, stand far enough away from support while leaning forward to complete 90° angle; head in line with arms, flat back. (5-30b) Drop chest forward and head down while partner gently presses down on shoulder blades. Hold for the stretch.

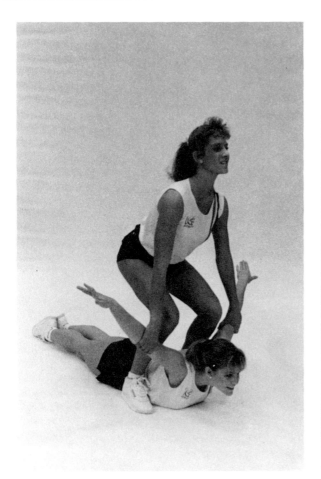

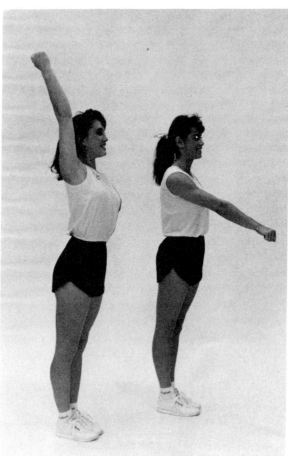

Figure 5-31   Figure 5-32

Figure 5-31. AIRPLANE. Lie flat on floor, face down, feet together, legs straight, arms out. Partner straddles with feet close to body knees bent, hands grip over elbows. Press hips down, lift head and shoulders up while partner gently pushes arms up and back. Hold for the stretch.

Figure 5-32. ARM CIRCLES. Standing straight, circle straight arms several times forward and backward. Extend circle to maximum range of motion.

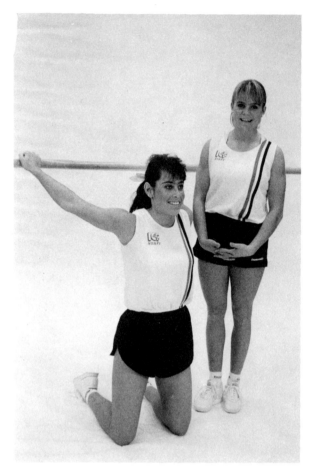

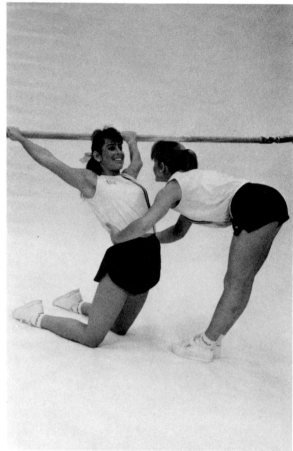

Figure 5-33a   Figure 5-33b

Figure 5-33a,b. WAIST PULL. (5-33a) Start on knees facing outward from bar or chair, or third partner; reach back and grab support. (5-33b) Partner grabs behind both sides of waist, gently pull out, hold for the stretch.

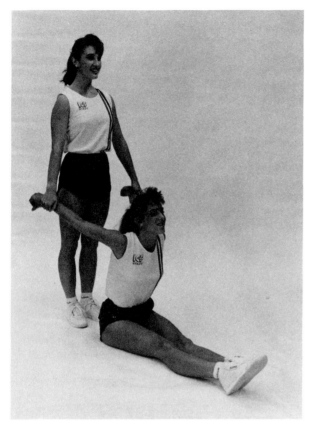

Figure 5-34

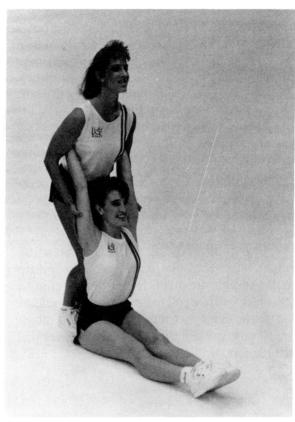

Figure 5-35

Figure 5-34. WISH BONE. Sit on floor in pike position arms back parallel to floor. Partner grasps wrist. Partner gently pulls wrist towards each other wrist. Hold for the stretch.

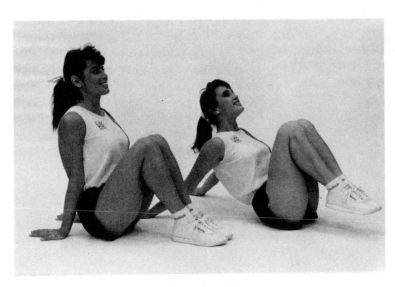

Figure 5-35. HYPER STRETCH. Sit on floor in pike position, arms extended over head. Partner stands behind, place hands on shoulders. Partner presses knees into back while hands press shoulders forward (causing hyperextension of shoulder girdle).

Figure 5-36. BOTTOM SLIDE. Sit on floor with knees together and bent upward, feet on floor, hands behind and close to body. Slide bottom forward away from hands (keep hand stationary); pull knees to chest.

Figure 5-36

Figure 5-37. WRIST ROLLS. With elbows stationary, slowly circle wrists several times in both directions; work toward maximum range of motion.

Figure 5-38. WRIST PRESS. Start on hands and knees, palms on floor, fingers toward knees. Keeping hands stationary and arms straight, shift weight backwards away from hands. Hold for the stretch (cheerleader on left). (Cheerleader on right) repeat exercise with palms up instead of down.

Figure 5-39. NECK ROLLS. Standing straight, hands on waist, feet apart. Slowly drop ear to shoulder then roll forward with chin to chest and continue roll to the opposite shoulder. Stop at shoulder and repeat in opposite direction. Repeat several times. Caution: Never roll head back in circular fashion.

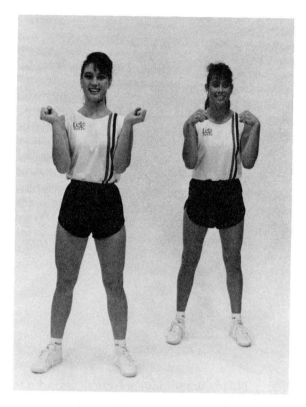

Figure 5-37

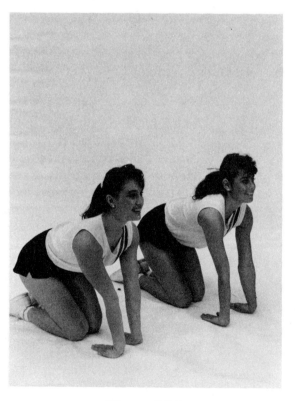

Figure 5-38

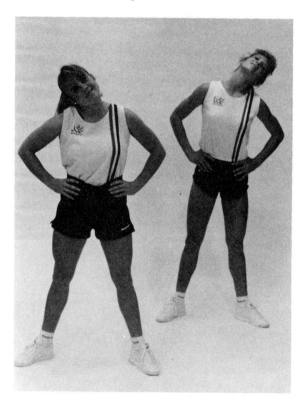

Figure 5-39

PSYCHOLOGICAL SKILLS

Chapter Six

Did you know that your performance can be dramatically improved or drastically hurt by the way you think? A conditioning program for peak performance must include psychological training because the way you THINK will improve your skills, increase your safety, and improve your overall poise and performance. "The goal of psychological training is to learn to consistently create the ideal mental climate that unleashes those physical skills which allow athletes to perform at their best" (Williams, 1986)

Imagine: at the same time you are spending hours practicing your cheering skills, the way you are thinking can actually be **undoing** what you are trying to accomplish! High achievers use their thoughts to assist them in accomplishing their goals; however, a "winning thought process" does not come naturally for most people. Developing mental skills requires training in goal-setting, controlling performance anxiety, increasing concentration and self-confidence. This chapter focuses on teaching you these skills so you can consistently perform at your peak each time you cheer.

THE BENEFITS OF MENTAL TRAINING

Mental training is a critical aspect of training and performance that is all too often overlooked. Picture one of your cheerleading practices. You spend most of your time working on cheers and physical skills, don't you? And no matter how hard you work, part of the time you just can't "get it together." This is when psychological training comes into play.

The mind and body need to be trained together in order to reach full performance potential and yet it is not often that you are taught how to <u>think</u> about a skill during the learning process. Remember, the way you learn and perform will improve faster and become more consistent when you have a solid mental training program as part of your workout. Coaches and cheerleaders alike often misinterpret the role of psychological training, in believing that only advanced athletes need this type of skill development. Mental skills training can, in fact, be beneficial for cheerleaders of any skill level and age group. **The greatest benefit will most likely be gained by cheerleaders who have the weakest psychological skills, such as lacking in confidence and emotional control.**

THE FIVE C's OF PEAK PERFORMANCE

Since mental training is a key ingredient of reaching your peak, let's learn how to do it! The first step is to determine which areas you need to improve and then design a program that will help you reach your goals. We have focused on five key areas of mental training — called the "5C's" — that will help your squad. The 5 C's are: commitment, calm, concentration, confidence and consistency. Let's examine how each of the 5 C's affect your squad's performance ability and safety.

COMMITMENT

What motivates you and your squad to stay with your workout program year round? The answer is to first **set goals** and then be **committed** to your goals. Commitment is the inner drive that gives you the will power or the motivation to stay with your program. Goal setting is one technique which has been shown to strongly influence athletic performance in a variety of ages and ability levels. In addition, it has been linked to positive changes in controlling anxiety, and increasing confidence and motivation.

You would be surprised how often cheerleaders think "I want to get better," but really don't have a plan to do so. When you set goals, you change the way you think about "getting better." Not only will you identify exactly what you are trying to accomplish, you will also know the steps it will take to make it happen. In short, goals change and maintain behavior. For example, if you wanted to weight 105 pounds by October 1st (need to lose ten pounds in six weeks), you will have to change your eating habits and exercise level (behavior). And, once you accomplish your goal, the positive feedback you receive will help you maintain your new behavior.

Table: 6-1
GOAL SETTING GUIDELINES
How to Plan Goals

1. Ideally, make goals **jointly** (coach, athlete and squad).
2. Identify specific goals in **measurable** terms.
3. Make sure goals are challenging yet achievable; difficult yet **realistic.**
4. Set **performance** goals as opposed to outcome goals.
5. Set goals for **practice** as well as for games, and competition.
6. Set **positive** goals.
7. See that each goal is **compatible** with your other goals and squad goals.
8. Put goals in **writing.**
9. **Prioritize** goals, focus on accomplishing the most important ones.

How to Accomplish Goals

1. Identify goal achievement **strategies** (how you will get it done).
2. Provide **motivation** and **support** for goals.
3. Set **short-range** as well as long-range goals and identify target dates for attaining each goal (i.e. new stunts).
4. **Evaluate** progress consistently.
5. Be **flexible** enough to allow for revision and change.
6. **Reinforce** goal achievement.

CALM

A cheerleader's success or failure as an athlete depends on the blending of physical ability, conditioning, training, mental preparation, and the ability to perform well under pressure. Worrying over your performance of a stunt that hasn't been going well in practice, or being uptight about cheering in front of hundreds of people for the first time, leads to performance anxiety. Getting a little nervous and "worked up" when you cheer is good to a point; however, when it turns into worry and anxiety, your performance will suffer. Unfortunately, worry doesn't just happen in your mind, your whole body worries.

Have you ever experienced that nervous feeling of "butterflies" in your stomach? How about your heart pounding, racing or "skipping a beat"? These physical signs or "cues" are associated with performance anxiety and the list is endless including fast breathing, increased blood pressure, the desire to urinate, muscle tension, trembling and twitches in muscles, flushed face, irritability, sense of fatigue, cotton mouth, cold, clammy hands and feet, visual and/or voice distortion, nausea, vomiting, or diarrhea!

Cheerleaders perform at their peak only when at their **optimal level of arousal.** As your arousal increases your performance will progressively increase **to a point.** Then, once your level of arousal goes beyond this point, you will begin to lose your concentration and confidence. You'll find you are holding tension in your muscles which leads to poor coordination, loss of speed and fluidity and an unnecessary drain of energy, such that fatigue is more likely to occur.

When you are experiencing more stress than you can successfully cope with, relaxation techniques can be used to get back on track. Try the progressive and quick relaxation techniques which follow during practice and performance. You **can** learn to control your level of arousal!

PROGESSIVE RELAXATION TECHNIQUE
(20-30 minutes)

Progressive Relaxation is the first step in learning the difference between muscle tension and relaxation. Use this technique during practice so that when you are cheering you will be able to use the Quick Relaxation Technique (explanation follows Progressive Relaxation). The progressive technique will help identify where you tend to hold tension. Your coach or one of your fellow cheerleaders should read the following in a soothing voice to the rest of the squad.

1. Sit (feet flat) or lie, arms and legs uncrossed, eyes closed.
2. For each of the following muscle groups, do a tense-relax exercise twice (i.e., tense hands, as though you were squeezing all the juice out of an orange, then relax). Allow about 5 seconds of tensing followed by 20 seconds of focusing on the sensations of relaxation. Then go on to the next muscle group.

3. **Muscle Area**

Muscle Area	Instructions
Hands	Clinch and slowly relax fists
Wrists	Bend hands back at wrist, relax
Upper Arm	Bend elbows, tense biceps, relax
Arms/Shoulders	Reach out in front of you as far as you can then relax
Forehead	Raise eyebrows, wrinkle forehead, then relax
Jaws	Clench jaws, relax
Tongue	Press tongue against roof of mouth, relax
Mouth	Press lips together, relax
Neck	Press head back, roll right, roll left, relax
Neck/Jaws	Press chin against chest, relax
Shoulders	Shrug shoulders up towards ears, relax
Chest	Take deep breath, hold 10 sec., slowly exhale
Abdomen	Tighten stomach muscles, relax
Back	Arch back, relax
Buttocks	Tighten buttocks, relax
Thighs	Straighten legs, tense thighs, relax
Legs	Press feet down in bottom of shoes, relax
Body	Scan entire body, if you feel tension **anywhere,** tense and relax that area again

QUICK RELAXATION TECHNIQUES

After you learn how to identify muscle tension (see the previous exercise), you will be able to use the Quick Relaxation Techniques described below. They are effective in dissipating tension and calming you down prior to and during performance.

BODY SCAN (5 minutes maximum)

This is a good technique to use shortly before performance or competition begins, or before practicing visualization of your performance.

A. Sit comfortably with eyes closed. Starting at your head and going down to your toes, scan your body for tension, and let it go. Breathe slowly and deeply.
B. Scan the following: Forehead and Eyes, Cheeks/Chin/Jaw, Neck, Shoulders, Upper Arms, Lower Arms, Chest, Stomach, Upper Back, Lower Back, Hips, Buttocks, Thighs, Lower Legs, Feet.

QUICK BODY SCAN (10-20 seconds)

Use this technique during performance, such as before a stunt or tumbling pass. Quickly scan your body in the same sequence as the 5 minute scan. Only stop at muscle groups where tension is too high, release tension, and continue scan.

NECK AND SHOULDER CHECK (10 seconds)

This technique should be used before or during performance. Feel tension in your neck: roll your head around your shoulders. Feel tension in shoulders: slump your shoulders.

ENERGIZING TECHNIQUES

There are times when you need to use energizing techniques to get motivated, especially when you are tired. Try the following energizing techniques:

BREATHING (10-30 seconds)

Focus on a regular, relaxed breathing rhythm. Consciously increase that rhythm and imagine that with each inhalation more energy is entering your body. With each exhalation, imagine letting go of any fatigue inside. Say to yourself while breathing: "energy in" and "fatigue out."

ENERGIZING CUE WORDS (5 seconds)

This technique may be used during a game when you need energy immediately. Associate energy with cue words you say to yourself such as "psych up!", "explode", "go!", etc.

CONCENTRATION

Concentration is basically "undivided attention." Although you may feel that you know how to concentrate, you probably have at one time or another not performed very well due to doing two things at one time. For instance, trying to focus on crowd rapport, game status, field conditions, etc. while simultaneously attempting a difficult skill. To achieve such a high level of concentration, you must be willing to **concentrate 100 percent in the present** and not think of past mistakes.

Next, you must learn to **focus your attention on the task at hand,** one thing at a time, and you must not allow yourself to be distracted. Finally, you must **practice concentrating** since this does not come natural for most people. The following concentration techniques will improve your ability to focus on and successfully complete your cheerleading skills in all situations.

CONCENTRATION CUE WORDS

During a game as well as in practice, discipline your mind to be undivided in attention, 100 percent in the here and now. Do not think about your date last night, or missing your last stunt. **Recognize when you are not concentrating and bring yourself back with a cue word that will trigger concentration:** "focus!", "think!", "here and now!", etc. One simple way to train yourself in this area is to have a partner who will hold you accountable for maintaining concentration throughout a game or practice. Begin by setting a goal of 15 minutes of quality concentration during practice and work your way up to the time required for a full game.

RELAXATION

By relaxing the body you calm the mind. Relaxing will help to clear your mind of distractions such as a negative crowd, frustration, anger, and a lack of confidence. Use the Body Scan, Quick Scan or the Neck and Shoulder Check techniques described earlier to relax your body and thus your mind during performance.

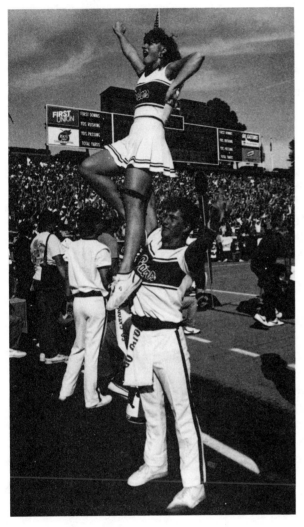

VISUALIZATION OR IMAGERY

When you feel yourself losing concentration, get back in the present through relaxation and by focusing on the appropriate image. Visualization will help you get rid of distractions, and focus on the here and now (see Visualization, described later in this chapter).

CONFIDENCE

Self-confidence and success are very much related. Confident athletes think they can and they do. They just don't give up. Typically characterized by positive self-talk, images and dreams, they imagine themselves winning and being successful. Self-esteem and confidence focus on success, rather than worrying about performing poorly or the negative consequences of failure.

SELF-TALK: THE KEY TO THOUGHT CONTROL

Whenever you think about something, you are in a sense talking to yourself. Positive self-talk can be a great aid to your performance and personal growth. On the other hand, negative self-talk is extremely detrimental to both your self-worth and performance. Your thoughts affect your self-concept, self-confidence, and eventually your behavior. Self-talk can be used to learn new skills, correct bad habits, prepare for performance, and build confidence and competence.

TECHNIQUE FOR CONTROLLING SELF-TALK
SELF-MONITORING: SELF-TALK LOG

The first step to control self-talk is to be aware of your own personal dialogue. Keep a daily diary for several days and write down thoughts and feelings, and what may have triggered them. You'll be surprised at **what you actually think!** Ask yourself: "What do I say to myself in practice? What do I think when I forget a motion or when my time is off during a squad cheer? What was I thinking when I finally got my back handspring or when I performed my best toe touch? Did I cut myself down when I messed up? Do I call myself names?" Pay attention to your thoughts so you can tell if they are heading you in a positive direction.

THOUGHT-STOPPAGE

Negative self-talk that leads to self-doubt and ultimately poor performance must stop . . . **now!** Learn to recognize negative thoughts; use a trigger word such as "stop", then change the negative thought to a positive one. Thought stoppage must be practiced, and it will take practice, especially when you are in the habit of thinking negatively. Change your self-defeating thoughts to self-enhancing thoughts and your performance will immediately begin to improve! It is called "PMA" — Positive Mental Attitude. Believe in yourself, argue with the negative thought, "Who says I can't?" Realize positive belief in yourself is a major step to reaching your peak performance.

CONFIDENCE HINTS

1. **Focus on the positive!** Pride yourself in the athletic abilities you have acquired through all the hours you spend working on cheerleading.
2. **Accept and learn from your mistakes,** then forget them. No one can tumble or perform stunts perfectly and there is nothing wrong with making mistakes. What is wrong is dwelling on the mistake, which leads to a loss in confidence and concentration, ultimately resulting in poor skill execution. Just **let it go!**
3. Replace every negative thought with a **positive** thought.
4. **Believe** you will achieve your goals.
5. Build a positive foundation. Tune in to all of the things you are good at, internalize the "winning feeling."
6. **Visualize** cheers, stunts, and tumbling passes successfully on a regular basis; see and feel each movement.
7. Practice controlling performance stress using calming and energizing techniques.
8. Work on your **concentration**, making sure your thoughts are focused on here and now. Visualize perfect execution of all parts of your routines (cheers, stunts, tumbling passes, etc.) prior to a performance.
9. The night before and directly prior to performing, visualize your previous peak performance. Recreate that winning feeling!

CONSISTENCY

Can you depend on yourself to perform consistently? Have you ever seen cheerleaders lose their concentration while they are performing? We all have seen someone "choke" in tryouts or in front of a large audience. Consistency is important as you perform especially because a cheerleading squad relies on teamwork. Try the visualization techniques which follow.

VISUALIZATION TECHNIQUES

Visualization or Imagery is mental rehearsal or the practice of rehearsing an activity in your mind's eye. Visualization is not simply mind over matter. A physiological effect of imagery is that it creates neural patterns in your brain cells and the more frequently you visualize, the deeper the pattern is. After a while you will perform as you visualize.

All athletes have the ability to improve their performance through mental imagery; however, just like any physical skill, it must be practiced on a regular basis!

VISUALIZATION TIPS
1. Before imagery training session, take 3-4 minutes to get completely **relaxed.** Prior to using visualization during the actual performance, do a Quick Body Scan and relax tense muscles.
2. Picture yourself performing a skill **perfectly** from start to finish as clearly as possible.
3. Visualize in the **same time frame** that it actually takes to perform the skill.
4. As you visualize, **feel** the action.
5. Use **all five senses,** become completely involved in the skill.

WHEN TO VISUALIZE
1. Every day outside of practice and performance time (10 minutes/day).
2. Immediately before performing a skill.
3. To perfect or make changes in skills you want to improve.
4. If you cannot physically practice, due to injury or sickness.
5. Regain a loss of concentration. Mentally execute your next skill.
6. Night before and morning of performance, visualize and relive your best previous performance in the environment of the upcoming event.

Commitment, Calm, Concentration, Confidence, and Consistency . . . where do you need work? Where are your weak points? What about your squad? The most important thing to remember is to identify the key areas you most need to improve in so you can plan how you are going to change your behavior.

Most psychologists agree that the ideal time to begin a psychological skills training program is during the off-season or pre-season. You are under less pressure at this time and you have more time to learn and practice the various mental skills. Similar to physical skill practice, mental skills training should continue as long as you participate in cheerleading! So go ahead . . . use your head and start winning!!

NUTRITION AND BODY COMPOSITION
Chapter Seven

> *"What is nutrition? Can it really affect my cheerleading ability?"*

As an athlete working towards being the best you can be, you are concerned with your basic fitness in strength, power, endurance, flexibility, and mental skills. The final aspect of conditioning and **one of your best tools in order to reach your athletic peak is your nutrition fitness.** The food you eat has a major impact on your health and well being. Your body uses food as a building block or a fuel for everything you do. Much like a car that runs poorly on a poor mixture of fuel, your body will not perform at its peak without a well-balanced mixture of foods.

Your dietary habits can definitely limit your cheerleading ability including crowd leadership, cheering skills, and overall performance. Good nutrition is essential because to a certain extent, you are a product of what you eat. The molecules and atoms in food are used to build and maintain your cells, tissues, and organs. A varied, well-balanced diet in adequate amounts will give you the nutritional basis needed for your body to function optimally.

Most athletes are constantly concerned about what to eat and what to avoid. The purpose of this chapter is to explain the essential facts of nutrition and their relationship to performance, weight control, and appearance. This information will help you make educated decisions about your dietary habits.

NUTRITIONAL BASICS

Nutrition is the study of the foods we eat and how the body uses them. All foods provide nutrients which are used to build, repair, and operate the body. Energy is provided by three basic classes of nutrients: proteins, carbohydrates, and fats. Minerals, vitamins, and water are also necessary for life.

PROTEIN

Proteins are your body's **basic building blocks.** They provide structure to your **bones, skin, muscle fibers and other tissues.** Protein is also the source of enzymes and hormones which control and regulate the chemical reactions within the body. The digestive process breaks proteins down into chain-like structures called **amino acids.** There are a total of 22 amino acids, 12 of which the body can produce on its own (called the non-essential amino acids), 8 essential amino acids which can only be obtained through dietary intake, and two that are inconvertible. The amino acids are then re-built into various compounds such as enzymes, hormones, and bones.

Contrary to popular belief, proteins are seldom used as a fuel source during exercise. The body prefers to use carbohydrates and/or fats for energy. Meat, fish, poultry, eggs, and milk are excellent sources of proteins as are nuts, peas, and beans. It is suggested that 15-20 percent of your daily caloric intake consist of protein.

CARBOHYDRATES

Carbohydrates are a major **source of energy** for muscular work. Carbohydrates are chemical compounds containing carbon, hydrogen, and oxygen, commonly referred to as sugars and starches. Breads, cereals, potatoes, beans, peas, fruits, flour products, and sugar are examples of carbohydrates.

Your digestive system breaks down carbohydrates into a form of sugar called **glucose.** Glucose serves as a major energy source for the body and can be found circulating in the blood (the blood sugar) or stored in the muscles and liver as glycogen. Stored liver glycogen, in addition to its role as an energy source, is also primarily responsible for maintaining the blood sugar at the proper level. Your central nervous system depends to a great extent on your blood sugar for functioning at its best, thus failure to maintain the blood sugar at or near the appropriate level can lead to symptoms typically associated with hypoglycemia (low blood sugar) including dizziness, partial blackout, nausea, and confusion.

The sugars that appear in our foods are classified as either **complex or simple carbohydrates.** The typical American diet includes several forms of carbohydrates ranging from common refined table sugar (sucrose), to the naturally occurring complex carbohydrates found in wheat, corn, peas, beans, etc. Since cheerleaders must be concerned with their athletic fitness, you should **limit the sucrose you eat** and **consume more of the carbohydrates found in products such as fruit (fructose), milk (lactose), and starches.** The complex carbohydrates do more than satisfy our "sweet tooth"; they supply us with many of the needed nutrients that make up a healthy, balanced diet. Approximately 55-60 percent of your caloric intake should be comprised of complex carbohydrates.

FATS

Pound for pound, fat provides more than twice as much energy as either carbohydrates or proteins. **Fatty acids,** the components which make up fats, are a **concentrated source of energy.** Fat is a necessary nutrient which provides not only energy, but also insulation and cell structure. Common sources of fat are meat, meat products, cheese, butter, margarine, mayonnaise, eggs, cooking and salad oils, cream, milk and nuts.

Not all fats are alike, however. There are two types of fats: **saturated** and **unsaturated.** Saturated fats are solid at room temperature and are found primarily in meat and meat products, whole milk, and butter. This type of fat can cause dangerous elevations in the blood cholesterol levels. **Cholesterol** is a waxy substance that has been shown to accumulate within the blood vessels and prohibit normal blood flow. Because of the potentially harmful nature of saturated fats, many nutritionists and physicians are recommending a decrease in saturated fat intake, substituting unsaturated fats in their place. Unsaturated fats are liquid at room temperature and are found in corn, soybean, safflower, and cotton seed oils.

It is recommended that your diet be no more than 30 percent fat, with no more than 10 percent of your fat intake being made up of saturated fats and the balance from non-animal, unsaturated sources. And, how many french fries did you eat this week?!!

MINERALS

Minerals are **inorganic compounds** found in small amounts in the tissues that are required for numerous vital functions. Calcium, phosphorus, potassium, iron, iodine, and sodium are a few of the most important minerals. Calcium, which combines with phosphorus to form your teeth and bones, is found in most dairy products. Iron, a key component of the oxygen carrying protein hemoglobin, can be obtained from many animal products, as can phosphorus. Sodium and potassium, which help to maintain the proper fluid balance in the body, are found in table salt and in many processed foods. Typically, mineral requirements are met simply by eating a carefully balanced diet.

VITAMINS

Vitamins are **organic substances** needed for the proper functioning of the muscles and nerves, for growth and development, and for energy production. Vitamins are classified as either **water-soluble** or **fat-soluble.** The water-soluble vitamins include vitamin C and the B-complex vitamins. Because these vitamins cannot be stored in the body, they must be obtained in our daily food intake. Vitamins A, D, E, and K, the fat-soluble vitamins, are stored with the liver or fatty tissues.

WATER

Since about 60 percent of your body is water, you must **maintain your fluid level** within normal limits. Water provides the medium for transporting nutrients, hormones, and for removing wastes, as well as playing a vital role in temperature regulation. Stop and think how much water you actually drink. Probably not much! You get the water you need from both drinking water and water in your foods.

NUTRITIONAL GUIDELINES
"I eat three meals a day, but I eat mostly the same foods.
Should I continue to do this or should I make some changes?"

BASICS FOR A NUTRITIOUS DIET

Food provides our bodies with the required nutrients for proper, efficient functioning. A sound, nutritious diet must be balanced with a variety of foods taken from several sources. This will allow for a proper mixture of proteins, carbohydrates, fats, minerals, vitamins, and fluids. The following is a list of seven basic categories of foods which, when eaten regularly, will promote optimal health, fitness, and performance.

THE SEVEN FOOD GROUPS

Milk and Milk Products (at least 2 servings daily). This group supplies calcium, Vitamins A, B-2 and B-12, a number of minerals, and a large quantity of protein. Low fat milk, when fortified with Vitamin D, is recommended. Cheese, yogurt and cottage cheese also belong to this group.

Breads, Cereals and Pasta (at least 2 servings daily). The body obtains its complex carbohydrates from this group which includes breads, cereals, whole grains, pasta, legumes, potatoes, and certain fruits. Protein, B-complex vitamins, Vitamin E, and iron are also found here.

Meat, Poultry, Fish, Eggs, Dried Beans, and Nuts (at least 2 servings daily). These food contribute large amounts of protein. Poultry and fish are lower in fat than red meats and therefore more desirable. Eggs are rich in all vitamins and minerals, but high in cholesterol. Liver is an excellent source of iron and vitamin A, but is also high in cholesterol. Vegetable proteins found in legumes and soybeans are sound sources of protein.

Butter and Margarine (at least one serving daily). Although high in calories and fat, these foods are rich sources of Vitamin A. Butter is particularly high in cholesterol and can be substituted with margarine high in polyunsaturated fats.

Citrus Fruit, Tomatoes, Raw Cabbage, and Salad Greens (at least one serving daily). Vitamin C is the most important nutrient found in this food group. Because the body cannot store vitamin C, it must be replenished daily. Lettuce and cabbage are not as high in vitamin C as are oranges, tangerines, grapefruits, and tomatoes.

Potatoes, other Vegetables, and Fruits (at least one serving daily). Potatoes, broccoli, green peppers, and cauliflower are important sources of vitamin C, minerals, some protein, and carbohydrates. Berries, cherries, peaches and other fruits are highly nutritious.

GOOD EATING HABITS

There is a major concern that young Americans (this includes cheerleaders) have decreased their consumption of complex carbohydrates and replaced them with fats and refined sugars. **These changes not only hurt your health, but also your cheerleading ability.** If you follow the nutrition guidelines we have just discussed, you will not have to worry about the quality of your diet. Your daily

selection (in moderation) from these food groups will help improve your health, appearance and overall cheerleading performance in the following ways:
1) Decrease your saturated fat and cholesterol intake.
2) Decrease your intake of refined simple sugars.
3) Reduce your chance of becoming overweight.
4) Improve your health, appearance and performance.

> ## FOOD AND ENERGY
> *"Everybody is concerned about calories, but I really don't understand the concept. What is a calorie and why all the worry?"*

CALORIES

The food we eat represents a form of energy called potential energy, which is released by the body and is eventually transformed into work and heat. Different foods contain a different amount of potential energy. Energy expenditure in the body and potential energy in food is measured in calories.

By definition, a calorie (also referred to as a kilocalorie) is the amount of energy needed to raise one kilogram of water one degree centigrade. Simply put, a calorie is a unit of energy. All foods have a certain caloric value and all activities have a specific caloric cost.

FOOD AND ACTIVITY

Your food requirements as an athlete are determined by two factors: 1) **nutritional needs** and 2) **caloric needs.** Eating a balanced diet ensures that no single nutrient will supply 100 percent of the caloric intake. The exact caloric requirement to successfully perform stunts, gymnastics, jumps, etc. will vary from person to person, but it is essentially dependent on age, sex, weight and degree of activity. Athletic activities require energy; however, among the many different sports and activities, there is a **wide variety in the amount of energy required** and in how fast that energy is needed. Anaerobic activities such as sprinting, jumping, weightlifting, and gymnastics require large amounts of energy to be expended in a very short period of time. Aerobic activities such as running and swimming, require large amounts of energy, but it is consumed over a longer period of time.

THREE ENERGY SYSTEMS

The body has three energy systems which can be used during activity. Two of them are generally used for anaerobic activities, while the third is used for lower intensity, higher duration aerobic events. There is overlap between the systems and very seldom does the body rely solely on one system.

ENERGY SOURCE #1

The first energy source is **anaerobic in nature and involves two energy rich compounds — ATP** (adenosine triphosphate) **and CP** (creatinine phosphate) — that are stored directly in the muscle tissue. Exercise causes the ATP and CP to break down and release energy for muscular work. Energy from these two inorganic compounds, however, is only available for brief periods because of the small amounts stored in the muscle.

ENERGY SOURCE #2

The second system involves the **breakdown of carbohydrates stored in the muscle and liver as glycogen.** Glycogen breakdown produces ATP, which when utilized in the absence of oxygen (anaerobic metabolism), creates a by-product called lactic acid. Lactic acid has been strongly associated with muscular fatigue and for this reason, this energy system is limited to activities that last approximately **one to two minutes**. The body is required to use oxygen to create energy — rich ATP if activity continued beyond this time period.

ENERGY SOURCE #3

The final energy source involves **using oxygen to produce energy from stored muscle and liver glycogen and body fats.** This is called aerobic metabolism. Unlike anaerobic activities which can be maintained for only a short period of time, aerobic activities can be continued considerably longer, primarily due to the use of oxygen which greatly inhibits the production of fatigue-inducing lactic acid and its ability to call upon the seemingly unlimited supply of stored body fat for energy. Aerobic activities are great activities for developing and maintaining cardiovascular fitness and reducing body weight.

FOOD AND BODY WEIGHT

"Losing weight has always been a problem for me. I know I need to drop a few pounds, but I don't know the best way to do it. Is there a good way to take weight off and keep it off?"

PRINCIPLES AND PROPERTIES

The basic principle underlying a safe and effective weight control program is that you can lose weight only through a negative caloric balance, produced when your caloric expenditure exceeds the calories you take in. The most effective way to create a caloric deficit is through a **combination of diet** (reduced caloric intake) and **exercise** (increased caloric expenditure).

OVERWEIGHT VERSUS OVERFAT

In determining your ideal body weight, it is more important to take into account how fat you are, rather than how much you weigh. Even though the standard height-weight tables have long been used to determine an ideal body weight, they are inadequate because they do not account for body composition. Many athletes, low in body fat but overly muscular, would be overweight according to these charts. These charts are based on generalized statistics and not on individualized body composition.

The best way to determine your ideal weight is to have your body composition assessed. This allows you to take into account not only what your total body weight is, but more importantly, what constitutes your body weight. Body composition allows us to divide the body into two components:

1) **Fat weight** or the accumulated fatty tissues in various parts of the body.
2) **Lean weight** (also called fat-free weight) which is primarily composed of muscle, bone, and organs systems.

Ideally, in male athletes the fat weight should not total more than 15 percent of the total body weight, and for females, no more than 20 percent. Remember, it is the proportion of fat tissue in the body — and not the bathroom scale — that determines if you are fat.

BODY COMPOSITION AND PERFORMANCE

There is good reason why an athletes fat percentage is lower and muscle mass is greater than it is for non-athletes. Fat cells and fatty tissues are not biochemically active in generating the energy-rich compound ATP (see earlier discussion). Thus, the excess fat contributes body weight, but does not function to produce movement. In physical activities that demand weight-bearing skills (walking, running, gymnastics, cheering, etc.), excess fat tissue is a hindrance to performance. On the other hand, fat free weight (FFW) is usually considered to be positively related to athletic performance because a large FFW means a larger muscle mass in relation to the total body weight and thus, a greater force potential.

EXERCISE AND WEIGHT CONTROL

As mentioned previously, the maintenance of your body weight depends on a balance between the energy (calories) you take in as fuel and energy (calories) you expend as fuel for your bodily processes and physical activity. In other words, **if you eat more calories than you burn, you will gain weight.**

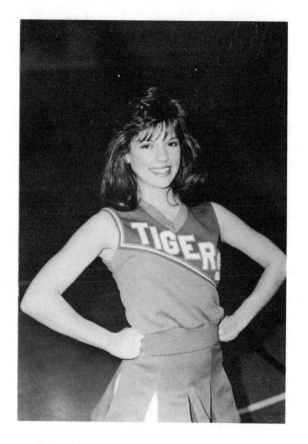

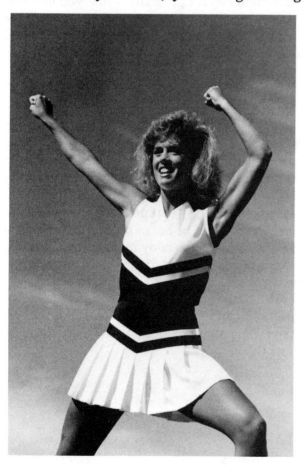

Conversely, if you burn more calories than you take in, you will lose weight.

ENERGY USED IN YOUR ACTIVITIES

The number of calories you burn during exercise depends for the most part on what you are doing. Not only do prolonged aerobic activities use more energy than do shorter anaerobic events, lower intensity aerobic activities will call upon the stored body fat as an energy source. Therefore, from a weight control point of view, aerobic activities such as jogging, swimming, skipping rope, and cycling (among others) will be most beneficial.

HOW TO LOSE FAT

Combine sound **nutritional habits** with regular **exercise** and you can sure of a safe, effective weight loss program. And, once you lose weight, this type of program can be easily modified to maintain your correct weight. Cheerleaders often try to simply "diet off the pounds" which is usually ineffective. Water is most of the weight loss — not fat — and this can also be harmful. Severe caloric restriction cannot realistically be maintained for more than a few days at best, and can dangerously alter the metabolic functioning of the body, potentially creating severe health problems.

The goal of your weight loss program should be to lose body fat, not muscle or water weight, and to keep it off. Fat loss is best achieved by setting realistic, attainable exercise and nutritional goals, thereby creating a negative caloric balance. Following good nutritional habits will ensure that the body is receiving the proper amount of energy it needs during the weight loss program, while exercise will help minimize the amount of muscle weight loss.

One pound of fat equals approximately 3500 calories; therefore, a caloric deficit of 3500 calories will add up to a one pound fat weight loss. Ideally, the total energy deficit should not exceed more than 100 calories per day. This is roughly the equivalent to jogging 3-4 miles (500 calorie expenditure) and cutting out a candy bar and soda pop (500 calories) from the diet. A 100 calorie per day deficit will produce a weekly energy deficit of 7000 calories which equates to a 2 pound weight loss (70000/ 3500=2 lbs.).

THE LIFETIME APPROACH

Some cheerleaders have trouble maintaining their proper weight and unfortunately, are faced with a lifetime "battle against the bulge." The vast majority of people include high caloric foods (especially fried foods, fats, and sugars) as a part of their regular diet. Combined with a lifestyle that is low in activity, this means very few people escape "creeping obesity" — the gradual addition of one or two pounds a year that, by the time we reach 50 years old, 35 to 40 pounds of fat have accumulated on the thighs, hips, buttocks, arms, and abdomen. The best defense is a lifestyle that provides regular activity and proper eating habits. The athletic diet and exercise program we follow while we are cheerleaders is a fantastic habit that will keep you in shape later in life.

DIETS AND WEIGHT LOSS PLANS TO AVOID

> *"Many of my friends have tried all the latest diets and have lost some weight, but the pounds always come back. Are there any effective quick loss plans available?"*

Have you ever known anyone who wanted to lose weight fast? The desire to lose weight quickly motivates many people to follow unsafe and nutritionally unsound "fad diets." Many **fad diets** promise quick weight loss, but ignore the importance of well-balanced meals and the role of exercise. Watch out for these diets as many have caused serious health problems.

For example, **low protein diets** may cause loss of muscle tissue and severe weakness. A **high-fat diet,** often times advocated in conjunction with a high protein, high fat diet with low carbohydrates, may produce kidney problems, dizziness, weakness, dehydration, irritability, and uric acid formation. **Low fat diets** lead to dry skin, constipation, irritability, stiff joints, and a number of other problems.

LOW CARBOHYDRATE DIETS

Low carbohydrate diets are the most common quick reducing diet, often called the "new and revolutionary" weight loss scheme. These diets cut the carbohydrate intake to very low levels while allowing you to eat as much protein and fat as you want.

When carbohydrate intake is low, muscle glycogen stores are depleted rapidly, resulting in fatigue. Also, for every gram of carbohydrate stored, there are three grams of water stored in the body. Thus, when glycogen stores are low, the loss of water leads to dramatic weight loss, but the primary component of the weight loss is water and not fat.

HIGH PROTEIN DIETS

High protein diets are popular among many athletes who want to build muscle and increase their energy supply, even though no scientific evidence exists which supports the use of these supplements. Protein intake exceeding the daily requirement cannot be stored in the body. Thus, the amino acids that make up the excess protein are converted to fat and the nitrogen is excreted in the urine.

"Super" protein diets are unnecessary, expensive, and in some cases, harmful. As for energy derived from protein, you burn as much protein watching TV as you do running at top speed. The body uses protein for energy only during starvation.

HIGH FAT DIETS

The unlimited consumption of fatty foods produces both health and performance risks. High fat intake increases the serum cholesterol level, particularly the undesirable LDL-cholesterol. Typically, high fat diets are high in calories, and since fat cannot be converted to glycogen, it is stored as adipose tissue and adds to any existing weight problem.

DIET FOODS

There is a widely held belief that certain foods will help you "lose" weight. Foods and food substances such as grapefruit, lecithin, safflower oil, Vitamin B-6, and vinegar have all been touted as foods that will burn up stored fat and play a role in weight reduction. Remember, all foods contain calories; therefore no food can serve as a weight reducer. Even diet foods have calories, although the number of calories have been reduced in comparison to similar products. Eating diet foods will not prevent you from gaining weight if you eat too much of them.

WEIGHT LOSS DRUGS

A number of drugs, both prescription and over-the-counter varieties, have been used as weight loss aids and to reduce appetite. These drugs, however, can have dangerous side effects and do not solve the primary problem of changing the eating behavior. No drug can take the place of healthy eating habits and regular exercise.

FASTING

For some people, abstaining from food altogether is easier than limiting their intake. Fasting, however, can cause serious health risks and should not be attempted as a means of weight loss. When you do not eat, your body is forced to draw upon stored reserves of carbohydrates, fats and, eventually, muscle tissue. The end result is a weight loss consisting primarily of water and less body mass with little fat loss, leaving the athlete weak, disoriented, irritable, and unable to optimally perform.

VEGETARIAN DIETS

Th primary concern with vegetarian diets is ensuring a sufficient protein intake. Most vegetarians are creative enough to meet their energy and nutritional needs as well as their protein requirements. Particular care should be used to select foods that will supply the body with the essential amino acids.

EATING AND EXERCISE

> *"I've heard a lot of different stories about what to eat before practice or games. What are the best pre-game meals?"*

Questions are often asked as to how much, what type, and the best time to eat prior to an athletic performance. Whether you are practicing or performing, it is best not to eat large quantities of foods less than two hours prior to activity. In general, cheerleaders should avoid the consumption of high fats, spicy, or foods which produce large quantities of gas before an event. Pre-activity meals should be light, fairly bland, consisting primarily of carbohydrates, and not highly salted or sweetened. A good rule of thumb is to avoid eating one and one half hours before high level activities and wait 20 to 30 minutes after finishing to eat again. Of course there are going to be many individual variations, but these are good guidelines to follow.

CAFFEINE AND SUGAR

Caffeine and sugar based products have the reputation of being "high energy foods." There is more myth than merit to the ergogenic (work enhancing) properties given to these foods, as each individual responds different to their effect. In general sugar and caffeine will not fulfill the energy requirements of an active individual and should be used in moderation, if at all.

DIET, EXERCISE AND WEIGHT LOSS MYTHS

Because so many people want to lose weight with little or no effort, product manufacturers are more than happy to oblige them by flooding the market with gadgets, diets, and schemes to "melt the pounds away." Beware of any product that boasts itself, as the "perfect, scientifically advanced, yet simple, way to lose weight." Chances are, it's a waste of money. Here's a list of worthless weight loss schemes you may run into:

1. Fad diets.
2. Body wraps, massage and fat suctioning — these are most commonly available in spas and questionable health care providers and should be avoided.
3. Spot reduction — there is no evidence that exercising a certain part of the body will remove the accumulated fat at that location (sit-ups will not reduce the spare tire and push-ups will not remove the flab from the back of the arms). However, as a result of performing these exercises, there will be an increase in muscular size and strength in these areas.
4. Steam rooms, saunas, and sweating — fat cannot be melted away regardless of what you may hear. Attempting to lose weight by dehydration is extremely dangerous and should never be attempted.
5. Weight training programs are considered to be ineffective for the reduction of body fat. In fact, resistance training is the preferred way of increasing the body weight.

EATING DISORDERS

> *"The thought of becoming anorexic or bulemic really scares me. Are they really as serious as they seem? What the the symptoms?"*

ANOREXIA NERVOSA

Cheerleaders beware! It is estimated that possibly one out of every two hundred adolescent girls suffers from this disorder which is characterized by self-induced starvation. Anorexia is a form of malnutrition that is very difficult to treat because the individual simply refuses to eat, primarily for psychological reasons.

Despite a skeleton-like appearance, **distorted attitudes** toward food, eating, weight loss, and exercise, **in the face of no other medical or psychiatric illness**, account for the extreme weight loss. Many of these individuals reportedly deny the existence of a problem. Anorexic females can also experience the cessation of menstruation and sometimes suffer a fatal electrolyte imbalance. Successful treatment consists of psychiatric as well as nutritional management.

BULEMIA

Another eating disorder commonly seen among adolescent girls is a "binge-purge" phenomenon called bulemia. Individuals with bulemia consume unrealistic quantities of food and then induce vomiting or take laxatives to purge the food from their body. Like anorexia nervosa, bulemia has a psychological origin. **Cheerleaders, bulemia is dangerous and can be fatal!**

Characteristics of bulemia include recurring episodes of binge eating — particularly in a short period of time, consumption of high calorie foods, unnecessarily secretive behavior concerning eating habits (often exiting the table to binge following a meal), repeated attempts to lose weight through the use of laxatives, vomiting or self-induced starvation, and severe weight fluctuations.

WHERE TO GO FROM HERE

The purpose of this chapter has been to provide all cheerleaders a sound basis for understanding the relationship between nutrition, weight control and exercise. A sound, nutritious, balanced diet combined with regular, vigorous exercise is the best strategy for successful weight control and optimal performance.

The goal of any weight loss program is not simply to take off pounds, but to take off fat and keep it off. Keep in mind that your body is made to be active and it thrives on movement and vigorous exercise. Regular activity, in combination with proper eating habits, will help you look, feel, and perform your best. Evaluate the way you eat! Get started feeding yourself right and before you know it, you'll be performing at your peak!

JUMPS
Chapter Eight

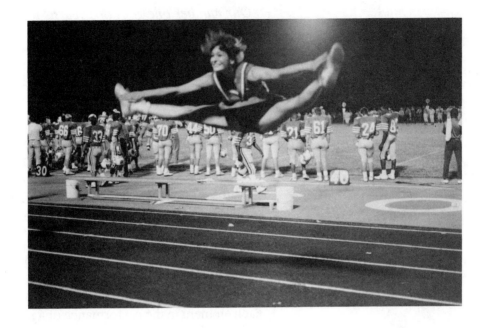

More than any other cheerleading skill, jumps are most closely associated with spirit and enthusiasm. To the average spectator jumps look impressive and the enthusiasm they represent can add much to your ability to capture your crowd's attention and support. Unfortunately, good jumps not only look difficult, they in fact are very demanding in terms of physical energy and precise execution. It only makes sense to develop the necessary conditioning which will improve our jump execution and our crowd rapport.

JUMP EXECUTION

> *"I'm confused. I never get a straight answer on exactly what should be emphasized for good jumps. Are there basic areas that must be work on to improve jumps?"*

Every cheerleader needs to master the four key elements of jump execution — approach, form, height, and landing — in order to perform dynamic jumps. Your **approach** or "prep" involves the explosive movement of your entire body that propels you into the air. **Form** involves the positioning of your body during a jump including the range of your arms and legs. The distance between your body and the ground while you are in the air constitutes the **height** of your jump. Your **landing** requires that you return your feet and legs to their original starting position. (Fig 8-2). A rebound from the flexed knee position is also included in correct jump landing technique.

If your goal is to condition properly so your jumps will improve, you must first determine that components of fitness (strength, power, flexibility, etc.) are necessary to emphasize in your workout. As we discussed in chapter two, applying the **principle of specificity** (exercise that mimics the activity) to your workout will help you see results. If you're going to spend the time and energy to train, then make it worthwhile by focusing on the four key elements of execution: approach, form, height, and landing.

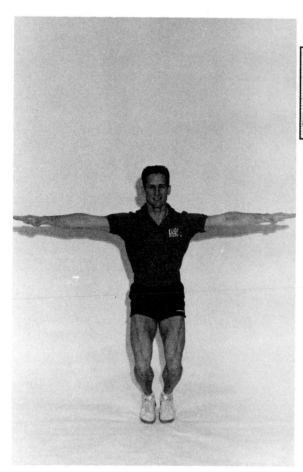

Figure 8-2: Jump Landing

CONDITIONING NEEDS

"Our number one goal this year is to improve our jumps. Since we have limited time for conditioning, what areas of fitness should we stress to make the best use of our workouts?"

STRENGTH, POWER AND FLEXIBILITY

Strength and power play critical roles in determining the height of your jumps and your flexibility to overcome the forces of gravity in executing a correct landing. **Flexibility,** both static and dynamic, is essential for proper jump form. In addition, flexibility plays an important role in reducing the incidence of jumping injuries, such as muscle strains. The use of **psychological skills** as an aid to the physical execution of jumps should not be underestimated. Your jumps can significantly increase when you visualize each element in the performance of a jump, as well as its overall execution.

ENDURANCE AND BODY COMPOSITION

Of secondary importance, but still having an effect on your jumps, are endurance and body composition. High levels of **muscular and cardiorespiratory endurance** will enhance your execution of a series of jumps and the performance of jumps near the end of a game. Remember, body composition affects the relative amount of functional tissue which is available for creating height in jumps. It may also influence the **range of motion** about a joint and the potential for joint injury.

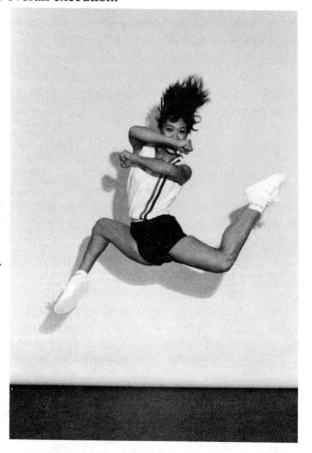

Figure 8-3

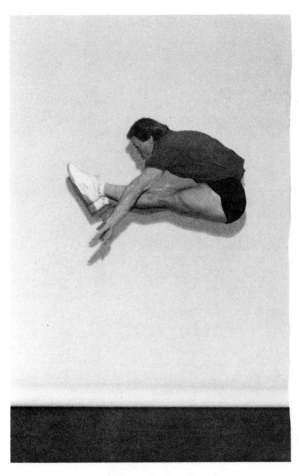

Figure 8-4: Pike

THE MUSCLES OF JUMPING

"Although I have advanced jumpers on my squad, I am often unable to point out specific weaknesses that are hindering improvement. How do I know the parts of the body that need conditioning?"

The last step in developing your conditioning program for jumps is to isolate the key areas of the body used in jumping and determine specific flexibility, strength and power, and endurance exercises for their conditioning. The following paragraphs describe the function of the primary muscle groups involved in jumping.

"We work on leg power at the end of every practice and I seem to have as much height as the other members of my squad, but my pike jumps never seem to make it to horizontal. Is there something I'm neglecting?"

HAMSTRINGS
(Jumps: Pike, Double 9, Herkie, Reach, Stag)
The muscles of the hamstring area (back portion of the upper leg) along with the buttocks (gluteals), provide for both hip extension (movement of the upper leg toward the back), and knee flexion (movement of the lower leg toward the back). Flexibility of the hamstrings is the principle factor which allows for the full range of hip flexion (movement of the upper leg to the chest) and knee extension (movement of the lower leg toward the chest) seen in a Pike (Fig. 8-4) or Double Nine jump. Strength and power in the knee flexors are used to create the bent leg positions in Herkie, Double Nine and Utah Reach jumps. Hip extension strength and power are important in lifting the rear leg of the Utah Reach and Stag jumps, as well as in the ability to return to the vertical position for many jump landings. In addition, hip extensors contribute to the power needed to achieve maximal jump height and to the forces necessary for a controlled jump landing.

"I've always been envious of cheerleaders whose jumps just seem to hang in the air forever. After working hard every day on my jumps, my form is much better, but I still don't have the height I want."

QUADRICEPS (Scissor, Herkie, Split, Double 9, Pike)
Hip flexion and **knee extension** are produced by the action of the quadricep muscles (located on the front side of the upper leg). Flexibility of the quadriceps is demonstrated in the full hip extension associated with the rear leg position of a Utah Scissor or Split jump. Strength and power of the hip flexor muscles are used to create leg lift in jumps such as the Herkie (Fig. 8-5), Double Nine and Pike, to name a few. In addition, the single largest determinant of jump height is the power-generating capabilities of the knee extensors. Another primary function of the hip flexors is to provide the eccentric forces (resisting gravity) which control landings (Fig. 8-2) and rebounding for consecutive jumps.

> *"Everyone tells me I have nice jumps. The only problem is that after all my hard work to get in the air, my landings honestly don't look much better than a graceful squat!"*

HIP ABDUCTORS/ADDUCTORS
(Spread, Toe Touch, Herkie)

The best example of **hip abductor** (movement of the leg away from the midline of the body) and **hip adductor** (movement of the leg toward the midline of the body) use is seen in the execution of a Spread Eagle jump (Fig. 8-4). To achieve maximal spread you must optimize your adductor flexibility and adductor strength and power. This cooperative interaction is also vital to the performance of Toe Touches and Herkies. Hip adduction plays a role in any jump which requires that the legs be returned to the midline of the body prior to landing.

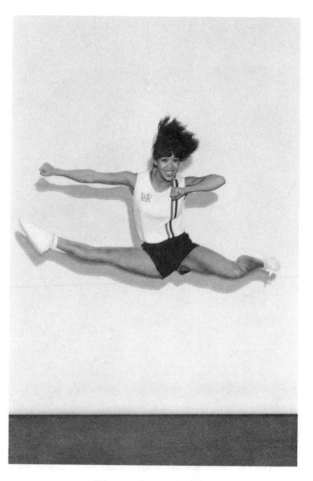

Figure 8-5: Herkie

CALVES (Reach, Double 9, Hurdler)

The muscles of the calf (back portion of the lower leg) serve three functions in jumping: 1) **Toe point** (plantar flexion) is created by the contraction of the gastrocnemius, soleus and plantaris. 2) Your calves are responsible for up to 15 percent of the **power** used to provide height in jumping and a small amount of the eccentric forces used for proper landing. 3) A small amount of **knee flexion** important in jumps such as the Utah Reach (Fig. 8-7) and Double Nine is provided by the calf muscles.

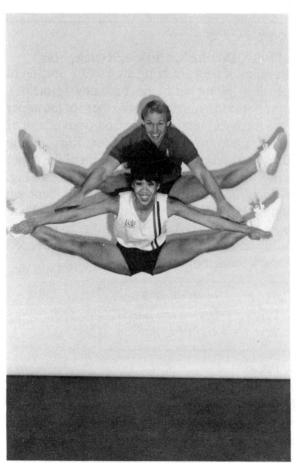

Figure 8-6: Toe Touch

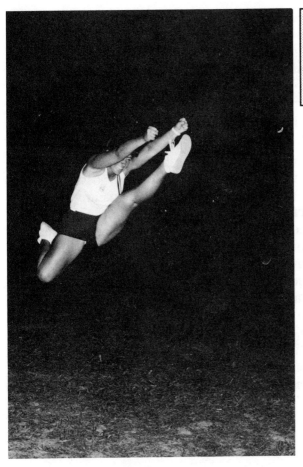

Figure 8-7

> *"My squad enjoys doing jumps as part of their chants. Unfortunately, some of them finish their jumps in a 'hunched-over' or 'squat' position and are unable to continue with the motions of the chant in time with the others."*

LOWER BACK (Double 9, Stag, "C")

Flexibility in the lower back is essential for maximal **trunk flexion** (forward motion of the torso about the hips) in jumps such as the Double Nine (Fig. 8-8 and 8-9). Lower back strength and power are used primary for **pelvic stabilization** (muscular isolation of the pelvis), thus providing the foundation for hips flexion/extension and allowing for the trunk extension (backward motion of the torso about the hips) necessary for upright landings. (Did you get all that?) Strength and power in this area, in conjunction with adequate abdominal flexibility, also contribute to the forces which create the arched back seen in the Stag and C jumps.

> *"Lately our squad has been working on getting our legs above horizontal in toe touches. We have the necessary flexibility and power, but when we really 'go for it', instead of our legs going up, our 'bottoms' go down!"*

ABDOMINALS (Pike, Toe Touch, Double 9)

Trunk flexion as performed in the execution of Pike, Toe Touch (Fig. 8-10) and Double Nine jumps is created by the abdominal muscles. In addition, the abdominals, along with the muscles of the lower back, provide **pelvic stability** about which the hip flexors/extensors and hip abductors/adductors can operate.

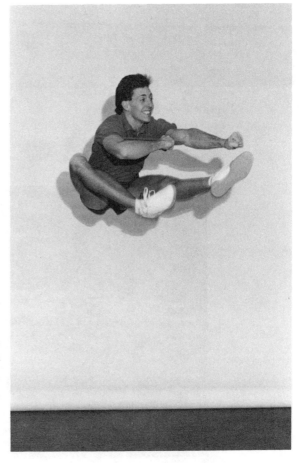

Figure 8-8: Double Nine

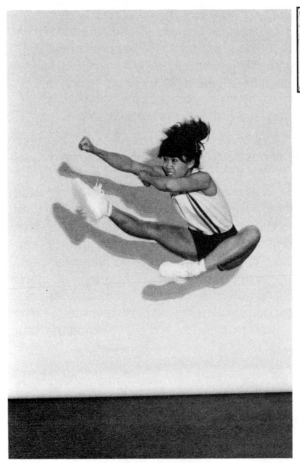

Figure 8-9: Double Nine

"I was a gymnast for several years before getting involved in cheerleading and I know I have adequate strength and power. I just don't seem to be able to use that power when I jump."

SHOULDERS

The multi-directional movement of the shoulder in the execution of a jump involves many muscles working together to create the most possible lift on the **approach**. The principle actions are **shoulder abduction** (movement of the upper arm away from the midline of the body) to achieve the vertical arm position, **shoulder adduction** (movement of the upper arm toward the midline of the body) and **shoulder flexion** (movement of the upper arm towards the head) to execute the arm motion, and shoulder extension to produce the upright position critical to a good landing. Flexibility and power through these ranges of motion are vital, because the proper use of the arms can contribute a great deal to both the overall height of your prep (Fig. 8-11) and the form of your jumps.

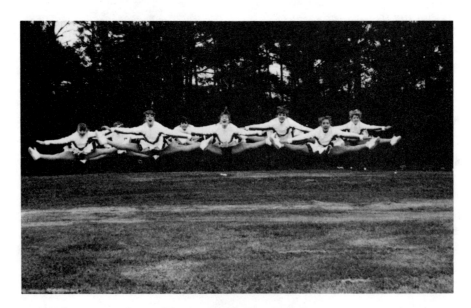

Figure 8-10: Toe Touch

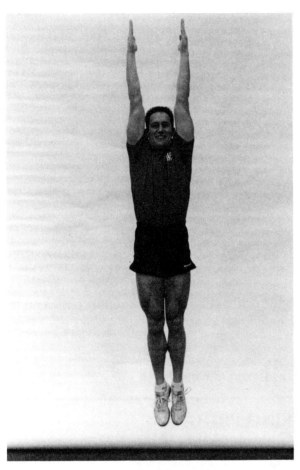

Figure 8-11: Jump Prep

PLYOMETRIC TRAINING

Plyometric exercises are an excellent means of developing the power necessary for the performance of cheerleading jumps and tumbling. Sometimes called **"jump training,"** these exercises require muscles to overcome the force of gravity exerted on the body during a jump landing. In addition, plyometric conditioning enables muscles to more effectively use the rebound elastic energy which is stored in muscles following jump landing. In short, conditioning through plyometric exercises will develop the explosive power and quickness necessary to create your best jumps and tumbling.

WALKING LUNGE

From the starting position take a large step forward so that the knee is directly over the toes. Keep head and chest up throughout the entire movement. Back leg may bend slightly depending upon flexibility, however, try to keep it as straight as possible. Push up and back off of front leg and bring the back leg forward driving knee up quickly and fully extend hip at the top. Go down slow and up fast. Return to starting position with opposite foot forward.

SWITCH LUNGE

Be sure you are warmed up and stretched out before attempting this exercise. Begin in the deep lunge position with hands on hips or comfortably hanging at your side. Keeping your chest up and eyes focused straight ahead, explode with both legs simultaneously, jumping us as high as possible. Switch legs quickly in mid-air so that you can land in a deep lunge position with the other leg forward.

DOUBLE SWITCH LUNGE

Elite cheerleaders can challenge themselves further by doing a Double Switch, where the legs switch front and back in mid-air, similar to a switch leap in gymnastics. Emphasize vertical explosion and rapid arm swing.

DOUBLE LEG BOUND

Begin the exercise from a half-squat stance. Arms down at the side, with shoulders over the knees. Keep the back straight and head up. Jump outward and upward, using the extension of the hops and forward thrusting movement of the arms. Try to attain maximum height and distance by fully straightening the body. Upon landing, resume the starting position and initiate the next bound. Emphasize "reaching for the sky" and the full range of hip extension.

ALTERNATE LEG BOUND

Assume comfortable stance with one foot slightly ahead of the other with arms relaxed at the sides. Begin by pushing off with the back leg, driving the knee to the chest and attempting to gain as much height and distance as possible before landing. Quickly extend outward with the driving foot. Swing arms in opposition or execute a double arm swing. Repeat the sequence (driving with the other leg) upon landing.

SINGLE LEG BOUND

Assume the same stance as in the alternate leg bound except that once a set begins, the opposite leg should be held in a stationary flexed position throughout the excercise. Begin the exercise as in the alternate leg bound but with one (the same) leg at a time.

DOUBLE LEG SPEED TUCK

(Note: speed tuck jumps are done on a resilient, flat surface such as grass or a wrestling mat). Assume upright stance. Begin by rapidly dipping down to the quarter-squat level and immediately explode upward. Drive the knees high toward the chest. Upon landing repeat the sequence, each time driving the knees upward toward the chest. Repetitions are performed rapidly with minimum contact on the ground. Emphasize speed of tuck and utilization of rebound elastic energy.

SINGLE LEG SPEED TUCK

Same as above using one leg, while the other remains flexed at waist level.

---

24 WEEK JUMP TRAINING PROGRAM

LEVEL	WEEK	SETS x REPS	LUNGES	BOUNDERS	SPEED TUCKS
Beginning	1-8	3 x 8-12	Walking	Double Leg	Double Leg
Intermediate	9-16	3 x 8-12	Switch	Alternate Leg	Single Leg
Advanced	17-24	3 x 8-12	Double Switch	Single Leg	Single Leg

Good luck as you condition for better jumps. Set your goals, plan your workout and be consistent. Before you know it, you'll see real improvement and it will be your turn to be asked the question, "how do you do those incredible jumps?".

GYMNASTICS
Chapter Nine

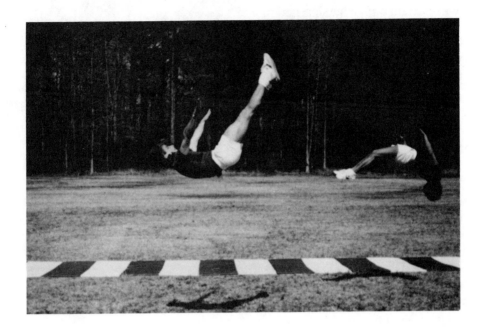

One of the physical skill areas that has caused cheerleading to become such a highly athletic and exciting activity is the increased incorporation of gymnastics. Along with a cheerleader's jumps, gymnastic or tumbling skills are one of the most important tools in generating enthusiasm and spirit within a crowd.

Imagine the point in a game when your team is losing and your crowd is somewhat quiet. All of a sudden the cheerleaders capture the audience's attention with a spirited, flawless back handspring series that leads into a favorite spirit-raising chant. Creating enthusiasm and keeping it going is part of your job as a cheerleader and the use of gymnastic skills are important spirit-raising tools. Gymnastics are not only fun to perform, they are also physically demanding and proper conditioning is a necessity!

What are the key elements of execution? What specific body parts are involved in gymnastics? Both of these questions will be answered in this chapter and we'll also discuss the overall importance of fitness as it relates to gymnastics in cheerleading.

ELEMENTS OF EXECUTION

> *"Everyone on our squad can do some gymnastics that we've taught ourselves, but even though we practice a lot we can't seem to improve."*

TECHNIQUE

The first key element of gymnastics execution is your technique. Using correct technique at any skill level is extremely important and, when learned in the developmental stages of your gymnastic skills, will build a strong foundation that opens the door for learning more advanced skills. Poor technique greatly **decreases** the chances of improvement.

Your technique training should include the **"prep"**, (Fig. 9-2) the actual **"rotation or flip"**, your **"landing"** and — for cheerleaders — the **"tag."** A "tag" is a cheerleader's finish to gymnastic skills which involves immediately focusing on the crowd and drawing spirit out of the crowd. It actually connects the skill with the purpose of raising the crowd's spirit versus simply showing off.

Higher level skills in gymnastics are based on a **logical and safe progression of the basic skills.** Learning correct gymnastic technique from a qualified gymnastic instructor is the most productive way to master the basic skills such as rolls and walkovers. Remember, in order to learn higher level skills correctly — skills such as back handsprings and somersaults — you must first learn the basics.

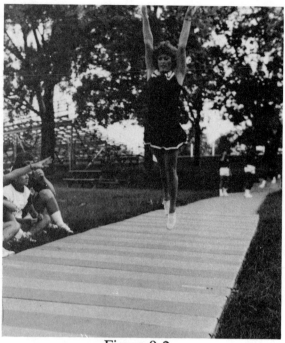

Figure 9-2

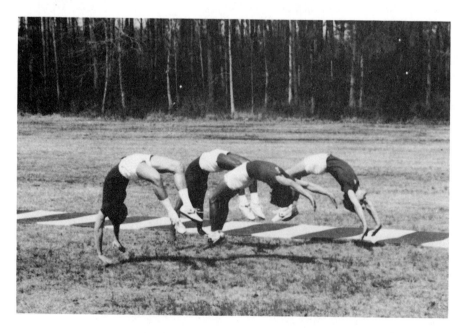

BODY AWARENESS

Body awareness, or **kinesthetic awareness**, is the second key element of execution. One of the most effective ways you will acquire body awareness is to develop a high level of concentration. Knowing exactly what each of your body parts are doing through a skill — specifically your limbs, trunks, and head — is a practical way for you to concentrate on body awareness.

Many times cheerleaders don't learn correct technique and body awareness; instead they are so concerned with just "making it over" that they completely forget about pointing toes, straightening legs, etc. Don't be satisfied with just "making it over" because this attitude definitely shows in your performance! Concentrate on knowing what each part of your body is supposed to do. Try to control your body when you perform the skill. This will make the difference between repeatedly practicing a skill and perfecting it.

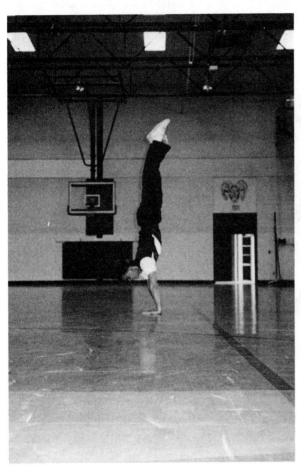

Figure 9-4

Although **lower level skills** may not seem to need much body awareness, this is not the case. Skills such as forward rolls look rather sloppy if you don't focus on the proper positioning of the legs and arms. Visualizing such things as the sitting position in the first phase of a back handspring being backward and not simply down and over can make the difference between success and failure in your execution. **Body awareness is a result of proper neuromuscular control.** Repetitive practice of a skill will enable you to know when to extend or flex a muscle group to produce the desired results.

BALANCE

The third element of execution, which is balance, occurs only when all **body parts are equally distributed and positioned over the base of support.** The base of support could be the feet, the hands, or even the seat. If one body part extends past the base, causing the center of gravity to shift, another body part must move equally and opposite in order to counterbalance.

Three exercises that will help develop balance are **V-seats** for the seat, **releve (on the toe) leg swings** for the feet and **hand stands** for the hands. To execute the V-sit — sit "Indian style," grasp inside heels, extend legs in high "V," hold. You can do the releve leg swing as follows: stand with your arms extended to the side, then raise your heels and balance on your toes keeping your body tight and erect. Lift one leg with support on the toes of the standing leg. While balancing on the toes of one foot, begin to swing the straight lifted leg forward and backward.

For **advanced balance work**, try to control a hand stand. (Fig. 9-4) Stand with the arms extended overhead, then swing your arms down to the floor while simultaneously kicking one leg, then the other into a handstand position. Balance should be controlled with your wrist and fingers. A variation of this would be to split your legs in the handstand position. Developing balance will greatly enhance your chances of success in gymnastics.

KEY ELEMENTS OF FITNESS FOR GYMNASTICS

> *"Some of my cheerleaders don't seem to have nearly as much power as others when they perform round-off back handsprings. Can this type of power be developed?"*

STRENGTH AND POWER

Cheerleaders must develop muscular strength so that **body control** can be achieved during the various activities they perform. Research shows that female cheerleaders have very weak shoulder girdles by nature; therefore, strength training should certainly be aimed toward the development of these muscles. Strength is also necessary in the **"trunk"** which is used for overall support. The **lower body is used in tumbling for "punching"** off the ground. This requires power training. Proper strength and power training is a tremendous asset to your overall fitness level and is especially important to the gymnast. (Note: "Overload principles" i.e. resistance other than body weight, are not recommended to children less than 13 or 14 years of age because of the chance of injury due to insufficient growth plate development.)

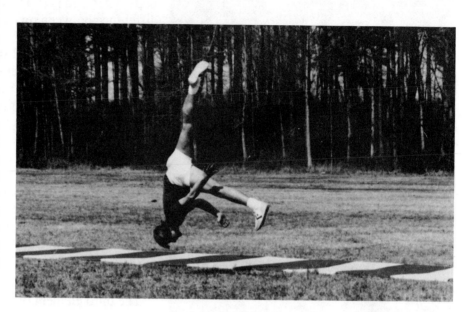

Figure 9-5

FLEXIBILITY

In order to perform most of the gymnastics skills involved in cheerleading, an efficient range of motion (ROM) of the major joints is essential. Flexibility is found commonly at a young age; however, you will not retain your flexibility without including stretching into your workout.

BODY COMPOSITION AND WEIGHT CONTROL

The third key element of fitness for gymnastics is weight control. Injuries can occur when a cheerleader has a weight problem. Attempts to perform gymnastics when you are overweight can bring about injuries such as shin splints and wrist and ankle tendonitis. Weight problems also restrict your cardiovascular fitness. Developing your tumbling skills — no matter what level — will be much easier if you first control your body fat. (See Chapter Seven.)

ENDURANCE

The final key element of fitness involved in gymnastics is your cardiorespiratory fitness. Your endurance fitness comes into play when attempting to perform tumbling skills successfully and safely near the end of a game or long performance. Your aerobic fitness (along with your overall fitness) is a key factor that allows you to cheer continually for an extended period of time and this includes incorporating gymnastics.

KEY AREAS TO CONDITION
(See Introduction for Muscle Diagram)

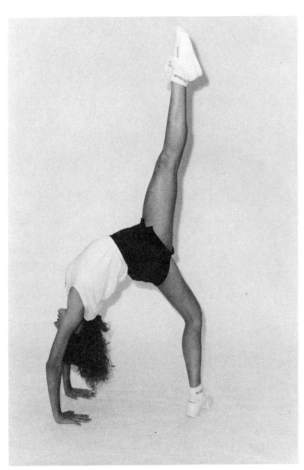

Figure 9-6

QUADRICEPS
Hip flexion and knee extension are produced by the action of the quadricep muscles. Flexibility of the quadricep is demonstrated in such skills as back or front walkovers. (Fig. 9-6) The strength and power from this muscle group are extremely important in such skills and aerial cartwheels and roundoffs.

HAMSTRINGS
The muscles of the hamstrings along with the gluteals (buttocks) provide for both hip extension and knee flexion. Flexibility of this muscle group is the principle factor which allows for the full range of hip flexion and knee extension seen in such skills as straddle forward rolls or the second phase of a back roll extension or round-off straddle jumps. (Fig. 9-7)

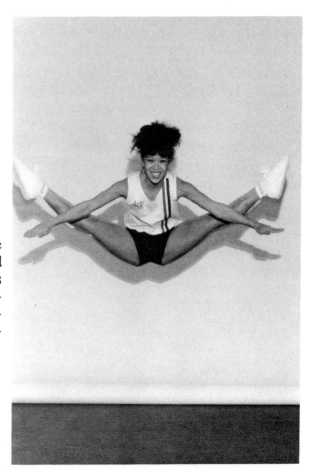

Figure 9-7

SHOULDERS
The most important actions of the shoulder girdle is abduction (pulling up or away) to vertical over head to block for repulsion. Strength in this key area is extremely important in such skills as front handsprings or mounters. Specific training of your anterior, posterior, and medial deltoid muscles will enhance the complete shoulder girdle strength.

ARMS

While the bicep of the arm is not to be neglected during training, the tricep group is the primary muscle group of the arm involved in tumbling due to its involvement in extending the arms. Strength gains here will increase performance during such skills as back handsprings. (Figure 9-8)

Before you attempt any gymnastics, make sure you know the correct technique to perform each skill. And if your goal is to reach your peak potential in your tumbling skills, your conditioning efforts will make the difference between average and awesome. It's your choice!

"If you fail to prepare, you are preparing to fail!"

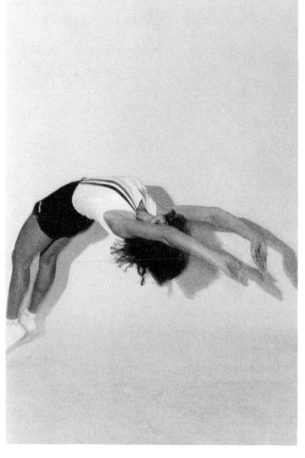

Figure 9-8

PARTNER STUNTS
Chapter Ten

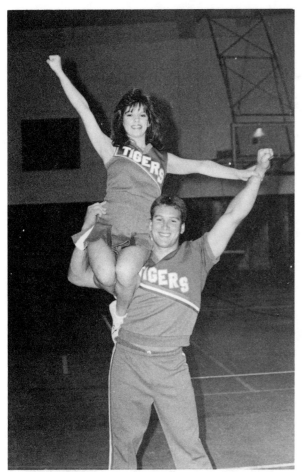

Performing partner stunts requires individual concentration and confidence, as well as good timing and body awareness between partners. A partner stunt executed with control and apparent effortlessness not only attracts a crowd's attention, it also frees us to focus our energy toward creating greater audience participation, as opposed to thinking solely about the performance of our stunt. The execution of all stunts demands general fitness, however conditioned athletes can more easily perform the high caliber partner stunts used in cheerleading today. The goal of a conditioning program for partner stunts is to provide the physical and mental abilities necessary to perform stunts safely, consistently and with apparent effortlessness.

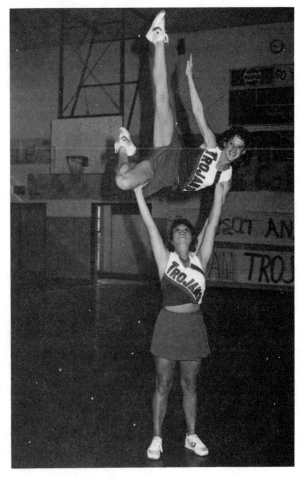

"Every stunt I learn seems so complex. Is there any way to simplify all there is to remember for each stunt?"

KEY ELEMENTS OF EXECUTION

The **proper execution** of a stunt can be divided into **three key phases**, each phase having specific responsibilities for the base (the bottom person supporting the stunt) and the mounter (the top person executing the stunt). The **preparation or "prep"** consists of the combined forces created by the base and the mounter which initiate the stunt. Another aspect of stunt execution is the **stability of the stunt.** As a stunt is performed, the stability depends on the body awareness and muscular control of both the mounter and the base. The final major area of concern in stunting is the dismount or completion of the stunt. The dismount utilizes a combination of the great forces required during the prep and the complete body control throughout the stunt to assure a safe and injury-free finish.

> *"Our squad's stunts are weak. We already have a conditioning program but we want to make sure we are doing the right type of exercises for stunts."*

KEY ELEMENTS OF FITNESS FOR PARTNER STUNTS

Look closely at the key phases of partner stunt performance that we have discussed. You can see that each element requires adequate **strength and power, muscular endurance and psychological skills.**

STRENGTH AND POWER

The primary function of the prep is to generate the large amount of power needed to transport the mounter from the starting position on the ground to the final stunt position. Both base and mounter use the lower body muscles to create the explosive lift necessary to put up the stunt. Upper body strength and power assists in the prep by providing additional force or "follow-through" to add to the power generated by the lower body. While upper body strength and power is the major factor in achieving a stable stunt on the part of the base, the mounter must use both upper and lower body strength to contribute to the stability of a stunt.

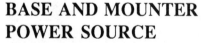

BASE AND MOUNTER POWER SOURCE

The base's primary source of power for the dismount is the lower body, with a small amount of force being contributed by the upper body follow-through. In contrast, the mounter uses upper and lower body strength almost equally during a dismount. As in the stability phase, the importance of muscular endurance increases in relations to the length of time a stunt is held prior to the dismount.

120

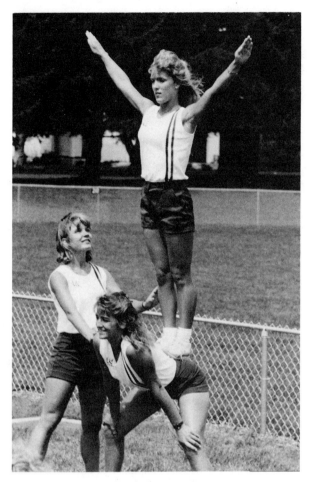

ENDURANCE

Muscular endurance is important for stability, especially when you must hold a stunt for a long period of time such as for kickoffs and player introductions. Strength, power and muscular endurance of the entire body contributes to the successful completion of a stunt by providing the final burst of force necessary for a safe, clean dismount.

PSYCHOLOGICAL SKILLS

As with other skills requiring timing and kinesthetic awareness (location of the body in space), good psychological skills are very important! Both the base and mounter must be able to concentrate and focus intensely on all three phases of a stunt. Both partners should visualize completing the stunt perfectly and work on confidence building techniques. The control of nervous energy can also make the difference between success and failure in a stunt.

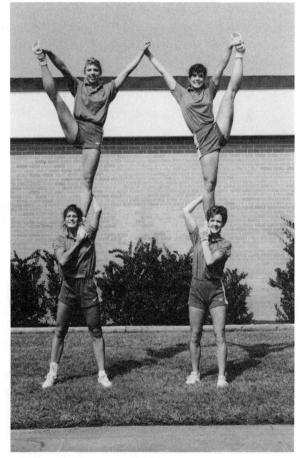

BODY COMPOSITION AND FLEXIBILITY

Though to a lesser degree, **body composition and flexibility** do contribute to the successful execution of partner stunts. Body composition affects the relative amount of functional (muscular) tissue being used to perform. This can determine the ease with which a stunt is performed and the level of difficulty you and your partners can attain. Flexibility comes into play when performing stunts such as a Star, a heel stretch (Fig. 10-5), a basket toss toe touch, or an L-Stand.

MUSCLES USED IN STUNTING

Most stunts involve key muscle groups which you need to emphasize when you condition in order to improve your stunting ability. In the following paragraphs we will take a look at the primary muscle groups for stunting.

Figure 10-5

> *"Whenever I base a stunt overhead for kickoffs or player introductions, my wrist strength seems to be the first to go. How can I increase my endurance for these stunts?"*

FOREARM

During the first step of a partner stunt — the "prep" — the base and mounter generate power through the forearms as they maintain contact with each other, transferring the energy of the prep into the lift. All "toss" or "pop" stunts use forearm strength and power to get the most height possible for the prep. Strength, power, and endurance of the muscles in the forearm help stabilize a stunt and provide once again for the transfer of energy from the base to the mounter needed for the dismount. Partner stunts such as Needles and Front Birds (Figure 10-6) demonstrate the use of muscular endurance in the forearm region.

> *"Our stunting ability is increasing rapidly and we've begun to use the cradle dismount in our advanced stunts. My major concern is whether we are strong enough to use this dismount for pyramids."*

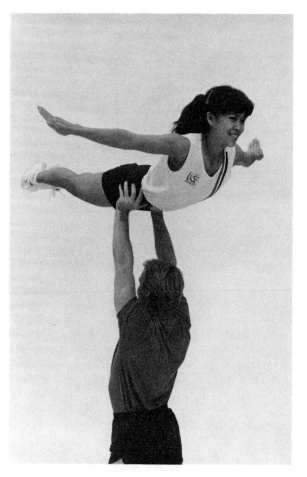

Figure 10-6

UPPER ARM

The **biceps and triceps** comprise the muscles of the upper arm. Strength and power of the biceps is used most often when dismounting. For example, the mounter and base use the biceps to support the cradle position commonly used to dismount from a stunt. In addition, the biceps are used by the base to create power during the **prep** as seen in a **basket toss** (Fig. 10-7) or a **"walk-in" extension.**

The **triceps** are used in all three phases of stunt performance (prep, stability, dismount) by both mounter and base. Strength and power of the triceps is necessary to create the final degree of lift in the prep, with the base and mounter using the triceps to "follow through" on the force created by the legs. A good example of this follow-through is a properly executed **shoulder-sit** originating with the mounter in front of the base. The **stability of a stunt** is closely related to the strength, power and endurance of the base's triceps. A few stunts also require the use of the triceps for stability on the part of the mounter as well. Holding stunts such as an **L-stand** or **Rear-axle** (Fig. 10-8) demonstrate the importance of endurance in the tricep muscles. The explosive power needed for dismounting, although primarily created by the lower body, also requires the follow-through of the triceps by both mounter and base.

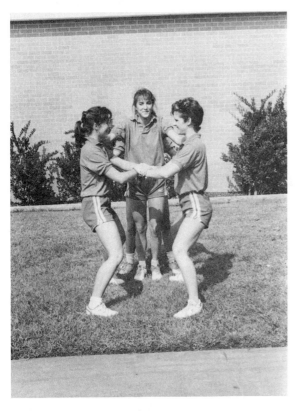

Figure 10-7a

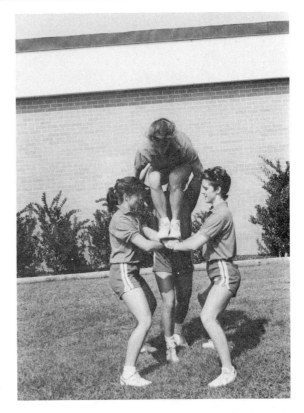

Figure 10-7b

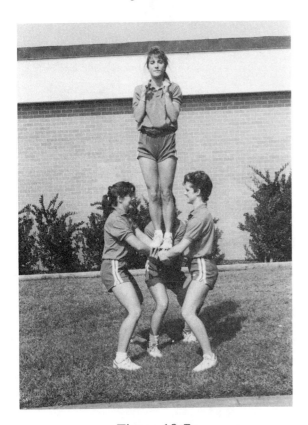

Figure 10-7c

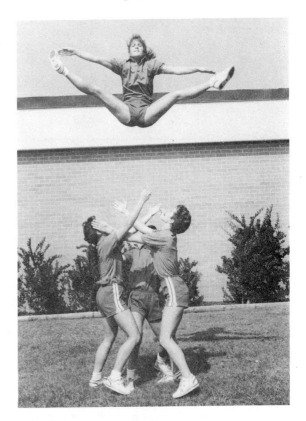

Figure 10-7d

"*My partner and I don't have trouble getting our stunts up, but they never seem to be stable or stay up very long. What can help our problem with stability?*"

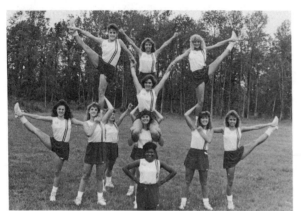
Figure 10-8

SHOULDERS

The principle muscles of the shoulder include the **deltoids, trapezius,** and the muscles of the **rotator cuff.** The strength, power and endurance of these muscles play a vital role in almost all stunts. Strength and power of the shoulders and triceps allow for the follow-through in the prep, while endurance of this muscle group is necessary for maintaining a stable stunt. Dismounts require strength and power of both the upper arm and the shoulder. An **extension** (Fig. 10-9) or a **liberty** is a good example of the complete use of the shoulder muscle strength, power and endurance, from prep to dismount.

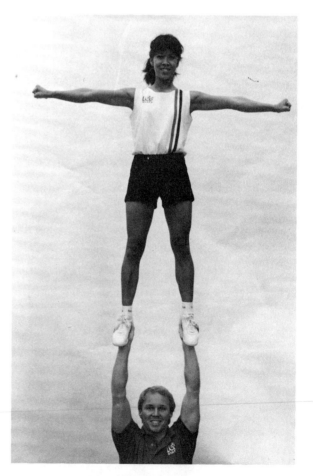
Figure 10-9: Extension

"*Every time our squad does shoulder stands, one of us ends up walking the stunt. Why does this happen?*"

LOW BACK

You might think that muscles in the lower back are not used much for partner stunts; however, they are used in almost every stunt! **Conditioning for strength, power and endurance of the lower back is critical to improve your stunts, and to reduce the potential for injuries.** The lower back muscles are used mainly to stabilize the spine and pelvis during each phase of stunt execution. They provide the base of support upon which other muscle groups create force. Adequate low back strength and power is essential for safe dismounting, while low back muscular endurance comes into play any time a stunt is held for extended periods of time. Stunts such as **Shoulder-stands** (Fig. 10-10) and **Extensions** demonstrate the great strength, power and endurance demands placed on these muscles.

> *"What cheerleading skills are improved by doing sit-ups?"*

ABDOMINALS

Newton's third law of physics states that every action must have an equal and opposite reaction. Therefore, creating muscle force for partner stunts requires that a **base of support** be established for the muscles to act upon. The abdominal muscles, along with the muscles of the low back, provide this base of support. They play a vital role in **isolating the pelvis** upon which the muscles of the lower body and trunk insert. The abdominal muscles also help the shoulder and arm muscles produce force by creating a "hydraulic cylinder effect." In other words, the increase in pressure within the chest cavity produces a base of support for the upper body muscles. This is similar to the base of support created for the muscles of the **trunk and lower body** through isolation of the pelvis.

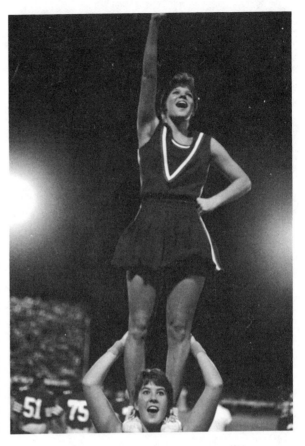

Figure 10-10: Shoulder Stand

Strength, power and endurance of the abdominal muscles is used by the base in all phases of stunting. For instance, think of how a base depends on the abdominal muscles to maintain upright posture when supporting an **L-stand** or **Sailor.** A mounter using abdominal strength, power and endurance is seen in a **Utah Reach** or **Side Chair** (Fig. 10-11). Finally, **cradle dismounts** require vigorous work by the abdominal muscles.

> *"Our squad recently added male cheerleaders. We really want to learn the 'toss or pop' stunts but never seem to get enough height. How can we increase the power in our prep?"*

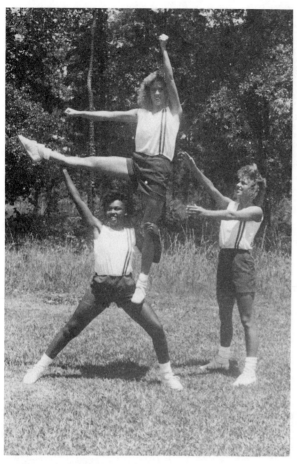

Figure 10-11: Side Chair

QUADRICEPS

The quadriceps include the muscles on the anterior aspect of the thigh which carry out hip flexion and knee extension. As previously noted in the jumps chapter, **these muscles collectively provide as much as 85 to 90 percent of your vertical lift.** It is easy to see the great role these muscles play in the forces created by the base and the mounter in the prep phase of a stunt. In addition, the quadriceps allow the base to achieve bone to bone connections in the lower body by producing full knee extension. This type of support is much more efficient than using muscular strength to stabilize and support stunts for long periods of time.

The quadriceps help both the base and mounter in dismounting. First, the quadriceps provide the mounter enough vertical lift to come free of their attachment to the base. This is especially important in stunts incorporating a **flipping or twisting dismount.** Resisting the forces of gravity (**eccentric contraction**) of the base's knee extensors allows controlled deceleration of a cradle dismount (Fig. 10-12). Hip flexion of the quadriceps allows a mounter to hit the **"pike position"** in a cradle. A mounter supporting her own weight in a dismount (by landing on her feet) is able to rebound by the eccentric contraction of the quadriceps.

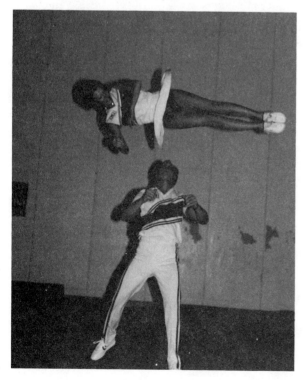

Figure 10-12a

126

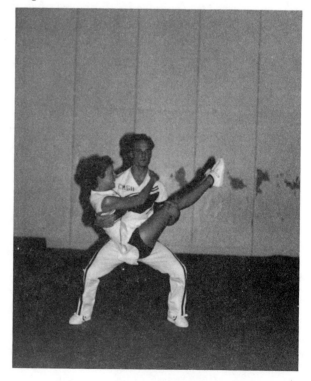

Figure 10-12b

MUSCULAR ENDURANCE

As previously discussed, muscular endurance is best developed by focusing on high number of repetitions, low number of sets and low amount of weight (see chapter 4). This can be done by alternating workout days, in conjunction with your strength and power program using super sets or circuit training (i.e. two sets for strength/power followed by two sets for endurance).

PSYCHOLOGICAL TRAINING

The way you condition yourself mentally will directly affect the success of your stunts. Any time you perform a skill that requires **timing and kinesthetic awareness** (location of the body in space), you are going to need good mental skills (see chapter 6). This includes being able to **concentrate** and focus on what you are doing, **visualize** successful performance, and **control your anxiety or nervous energy.** Your squad should not attempt any partner stunts until everyone understands that mental skills can make the difference whether you succeed or fail in a stunt.

Partner stunts are one of the most exciting aspects of cheerleading today. With a good plan and hard work, you can improve your stunts and be on your way to exciting your crowd like never before. Conditioning is the key.

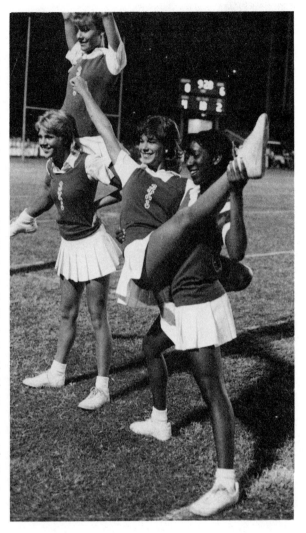

DANCE
Chapter Eleven

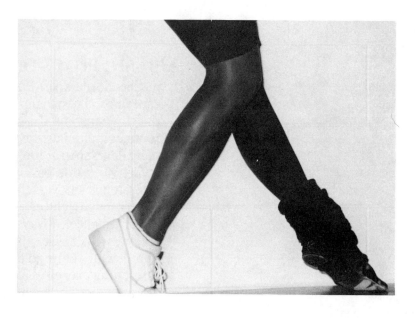

Nothing is more dynamic than the spark of a dance routine performed by a cheerleading squad to exciting music! Dance has always been an excellent means of entertainment and a sure way to generate spirit and excitement. With the increasing popularity of dance in cheerleading, we are seeing many different styles emerging and more men becoming involved. Whether your squad is "drill" or "funky", there are definite basic techniques for all styles and, believe it or not, conditioning for dance is just as important as it is for jumps, partner stunts, and other cheerleading skills.

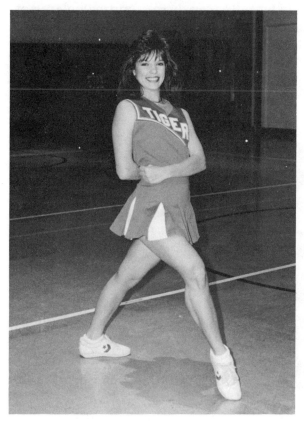

KEY ELEMENTS OF FITNESS

Dance cannot be learned overnight, but through proper conditioning combined with learning basic dance exercises and skills, you can become more proficient. For example, the more flexible you are, the higher you can kick, providing you have the right amount of strength. Because of the tremendous amount of variety in dance movement, an **overall conditioning program stressing strength, power, flexibility, and endurance will help you most in developing dynamic cheerleading dance skills.**

Being in better shape will increase the number of movements you can learn and perform effectively. Stretching and strengthening your muscles and concentrating on good alignment will improve your execution of turns, kicks, jumps and lunges. Isolation and improvisation techniques increase body awareness. Psychological skills are especially important in dance as they affect your ability to project enthusiasm and excitement to your audience. Finally, good cardiorespiratory conditioning will increase your stamina, allowing you to perform your routines in an energetic, spirited manner and hopefully, you'll even be able to keep that smile on your face!

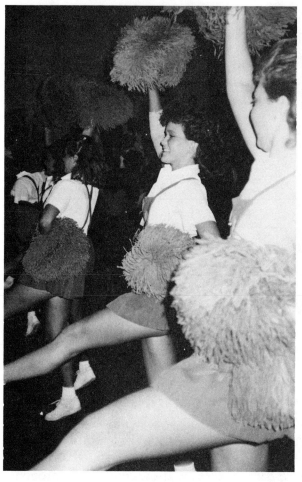

KEY ELEMENTS OF DANCE

"After performing several pom routines, my legs are killing me! What am I doing wrong?"

BASIC POM STEPS

Cheerleaders perform many different types of dance, especially the standard "fight song type" pom routines. There are basic elements common to pom routines including a fast, energetic "Pom Step" (originally developed as the "Bruin High Step"). Although styles vary, this basic step involves an alternating "step-touch" movement (step on right, touch left, step on left, touch right, etc.). If your pom step includes the use of your heel, always land **toe-ball-heel** as you step (Figures 11-00A-c). If your style does not require your heel to return to the surface, be sure to perform **stretching exercises** for your calf muscles before and after practices or a game.

Both **cardiorespiratory** and **muscular endurance** are necessary to continuously perform pom routines. To develop the muscular endurance needed for a game, practice the pom step over increasing periods of time. You can also perform multiple sets of calf raises. A good aerobic workout will help build your stamina to practice routines continuously and to perform long routines. **To avoid overuse injuries** (i.e. shin splits), incorporate proper stretching and strengthening of your lower leg muscles in your workout. Also, make sure your cheerleading shoes have adequate padding (effective shock absorption) at the ball of the foot.

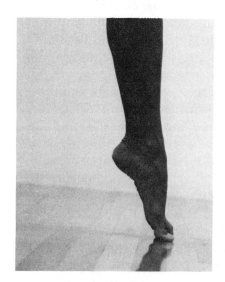

Figure 11-00A

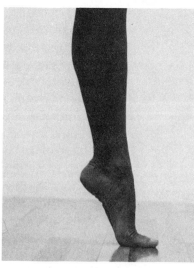

Figure 11-00B

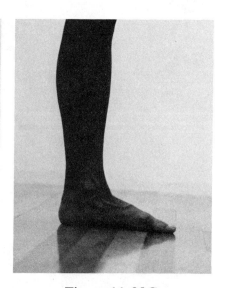

Figure 11-00C

> *"The dances we learn in cheerleading seem to require lots of wide straddle positions and deep lunges. Is there a way to condition for these?"*

STANCES AND LUNGES

Lunges can either be performed forward or to the side. **There are two major sets of muscles involved in the lunge — one located about the knee joint, the other around the hip joint.** The muscles around the knee joint are the quadriceps femoris muscle group. In the hip joint the major muscles used are the hip flexors in front and gluteus maximus and the hamstring group behind. When you execute a lunge, it is essential that your trunk remain erect. If you are performing a dance movement while in a lunge — for example, a body wave— keep your pelvic area stable and wave only with the upper body. With the trunk in this position, maximum flexion in the hip joint of the forward leg occurs; which in turn requires maximum force in the gluteus maximus muscle. In other words, **the deeper your lunge, the greater the use of the gluteus maximus and hamstring muscles, and the greater the hip-joint flexibility needed.** Be careful not to place too much stress on your knee by doing a bend that is too deep.

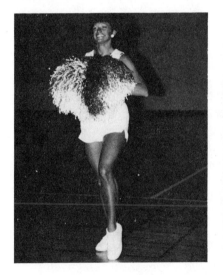
Figure 11-4A

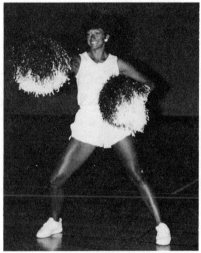
Figure 11-4B

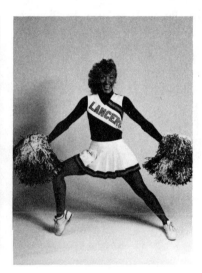
Figure 11-5

Points to remember:
1. Hold abdominals in, keeping torso erect and hips square.
2. Lunge forward or to the side, with the lower leg perpendicular to floor (i.e. knee over heel).
3. Keep rear (or side) leg bent to isolate the buttocks and avoid hyperextension of the knee.
4. Avoid lunging too deeply to prevent knee strain.

TURNS AND ALIGNMENT

Cheerleaders often lose their balance performing turns in dance routines. This is because an arched back and expanded rip cage invariably result in a spiral effect which will cause you to lose your balance. In order to correct this, let's look at **the most important basic principle of dance — alignment.**

It is beyond the scope of this book to discuss individual alignment problems such as lordosis, scoliosis and kyphosis, but it is important that cheerleaders strive for what is called **"center"** in dance. It is the balance point you always must reach for in order to improve the execution of your turns, kicks, and dance steps. Not only does it aid in turns, it decreases the chance of getting injured in the joint areas or the lower back.

To achieve proper alignment for dancing, your back is allowed only its natural curve, with your stomach muscles pulled in and upward. In addition, the ribs are closed, the chest is lifted and the shoulders are pulled gently down and back. The feeling of length and elasticity must extend all the way through to the top of your head by stretching the back of your neck. The sooner this position becomes automatic for you, the better you will perform! (An exception to this placement is necessary when performing a leap or jump specifically requiring an arch, such as a "C" jump which uses the arch to bring the back foot to the head.)

It is important to note that this positioning should not only be practiced in turns, but in the basic stance position used by many cheerleading squads. **In a basic stance, your feet should be parallel and wider than your shoulders with your knees always in alignment with your feet and toes.** Calf muscle strength is also important as you must stay on your toes to execute a good turn. The flexing and pointing of the supporting foot must be felt, so that you are not sagging or sitting into the turn.

Exercises for good alignment always should include strengthening your abdominals and upper back. (Fig. 11-6) Calf muscles should also be strengthened for turns. **Flexibility stretches** should focus on these areas: calves, hamstrings, quadriceps, hip flexors, anterior chest, and lower back. Unfortunately, even with the best conditioning, good turns cannot be performed without solid technique, so concentrate on the proper presentation, arm carriage and "spotting" (focusing with your eyes, as well as your head) to control your turns.

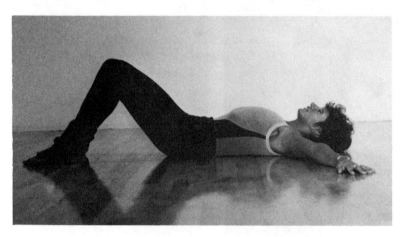

Figure 11-6A

"When the cheerleaders on my squad perform routines with high kicks, we never look good because some of us kick really high and others don't. Are there exercises we can do so we all will have high kicks?"

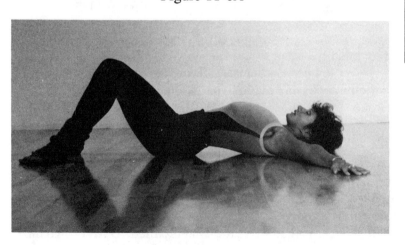

Figure 11-6B

KICKS

High kicks are one of the most visible parts of your dance routines. Proper execution of a front, side and back kick requires brushing the floor with a pointed toe (tendu), lifting the leg as high as possible and returning the leg to its original position. All this requires good **strength and flexibility.** Of course, the more flexible you are, the greater your range of motion, and thus, the higher your kick. But you must also have the necessary strength to get your leg in the air. Increasing your quadriceps and hip abductor strength will help with your front and side kicks. (Fig. 11-7) Increasing your hamstring strength will assist with your back leg kicks. Remember that proper technique for a side kick (Fig. 11-8) requires that the knee be facing up during the execution of the kick and thus you are using the quadriceps muscles more than the hip abductors.

To increase your flexibility, hold the front and side split position on the ground for 30 to 60 seconds. By lying on your back and kicking your leg straight up in front of you approximately 20-25 times you can **increase your muscular endurance for front kicks.** Remember to practice the leg kicks while lying on your side with your knee facing up so as to exactly duplicate what you will be doing when standing. Gravity will assist in bringing your leg down unless you move immediately into another position. And of course, always keep the rest of your body in good alignment, so as not to cause injury to your knee or hip joints.

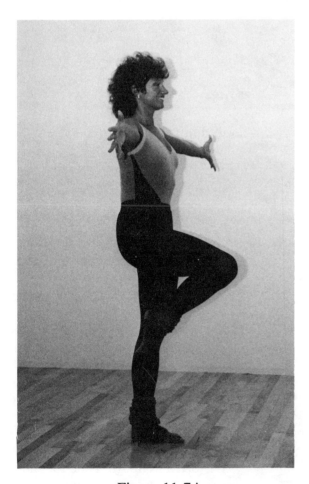

Figure 11-7A

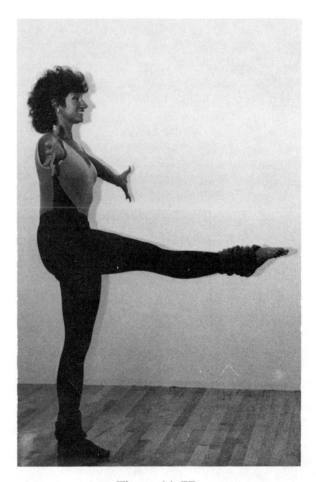

Figure 11-7B

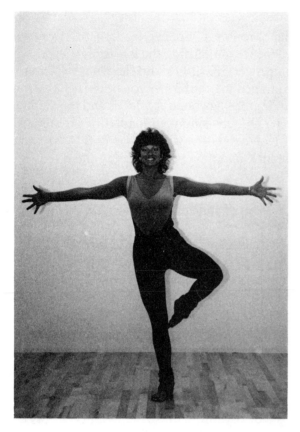

Figure 11-8A

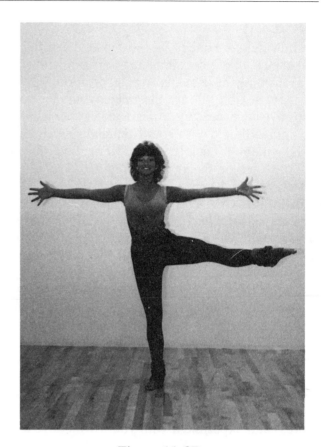

Figure 11-8B

> *"The jumps we use in dance routines are different from those we use to cheer. Is the conditioning different?"*

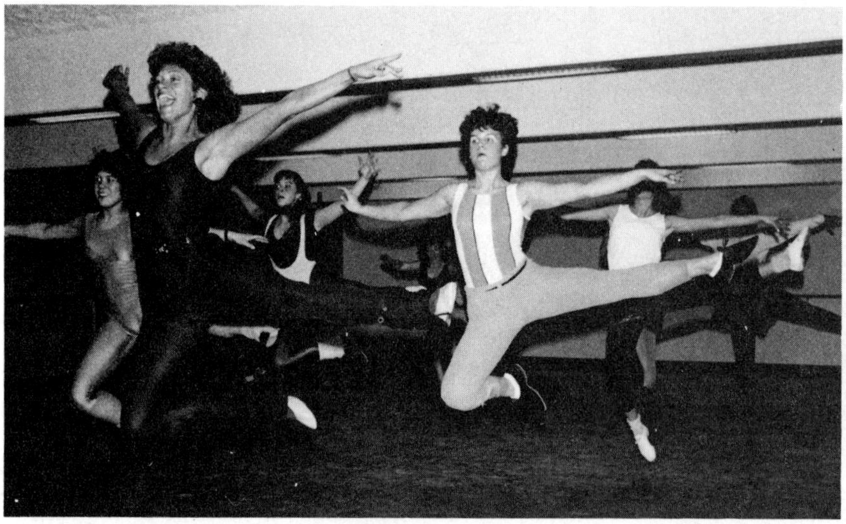

JUMPS AND LEAPS

The key elements of execution and fitness are the same for cheerleading jumps (see chapter eight) as they are for dance jumps; however, there is one importance difference. **Dance jumps/leaps often take off from one foot, as opposed to the two foot preparation used in jumps such as a toe touch or a herkie.** For example, the back leg in a stag or split jump originating from one foot must kick backward vigorously by using a strong digging thrust into the ground and by quick

Figure 11-9

contraction of the buttock and back muscles. Incorporating leg lifts (quick) into your conditioning program can be done to exercise muscles in the groin which contract to lift the front leg horizontally forward. In a dance routine, you may land in various positions, therefore, an overall muscle strength and conditioning program is necessary to develop more **control in the air and when landing.**

> *"My squad has always done pom routines but we now are using dance in our half time cheer routines. Some of the cheerleaders look too stiff. Is is possible to work on 'loosening up'?"*

ISOLATIONS AND RHYTHM

Isolation exercises are great for developing body awareness (i.e. kinesthetic awareness). You can perform an isolation exercise by exercising one specific part of your body while trying not to move anything else. Try isolating just your head in a forward and backward or side to side movement (use caution and always avoid sharp head movements backward). Next, isolate your shoulders by lifting them up and down individually or together. The rib cage is the biggest challenge. Move your rib cage side to side or front to back without collapsing your chest. (It's not easy, is it?) Hips are probably used the most, so practice moving your hips in all directions without moving any other part of your body. Continue trying different areas of your body such as the knees, legs and arms to different tempos of music. Even though you are trying to isolate, do not overlook the fact that every part of the body has a connection to and a relationship with other parts of the body.

Obviously, **rhythm is something for which you cannot condition,** but to develop more body awareness try **improvisation.** Subconscious related improvisation is the best way to learn how to relax and "let go." It means to compose or invent on the spur of the moment. Improvisation is a chance to express and experiment with your own body, with music or rhythm, with space, with concepts and emotions. Go to a room or studio alone, turn on some music and let your body go! Occasionally envision an audience and try to create for them. This procedure when done correctly allows your subconscious to operate. One final note, **remember to choreograph to fit your squad rather than fitting your squad to choreography.**

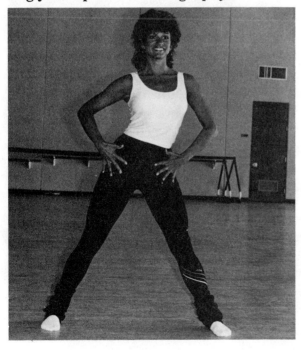

Figure 11-10

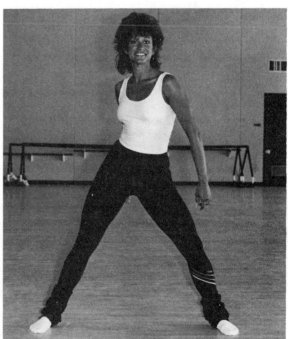

Figure 11-11

> *"Cheerleading is always strenuous but when we do our dances, everybody gets tired. What should we do?"*

CARDIORESPIRATORY ENDURANCE

Good cardiorespiratory endurance is important in all phases of cheerleading; however, it is essential in dance. Your squad needs a lot of stamina to cheer continuously throughout a game and still be able to perform a dance routine or fight song effectively. Whether it's running, biking, jumping rope or — as mentioned earlier in the pom step section — repeating a dance routine consistently a number of times, you must try to raise your heart rate to training threshold for 15-20 minutes at least three times per week. Several good ideas for endurance training can be found in chapter three.

> *"Our squad dances a lot and I think my knees are weak because they always begin hurting at the start of our cheerleading season. Is there anything I can do to help them?"*

MUSCLE ENDURANCE

KNEES

Dance moves uses space, different levels, accents, and rhythm changes that put stress on knees. Correct alignment of the knee in relationship to the thigh and lower leg will rarely result in any chronic strain. In most injuries, the problem arises from improper positioning of the leg while in the bent knee position. **The best way to support your knees is to be sure your hamstrings and quadriceps are in a 2 to 3 strength ratio.** That is, the amount of force produced during knee flexion should be approximately 67 percent of the force produced during knee extension. One final caution: Knee drops should either be avoided completely or performed cautiously with hands touching the ground first to break your fall.

ARMS

The technique and conditioning for your arms is equally important as for your legs. For muscular endurance, practice movements that are similar to the cheerleading routine movements. By using light hand weights in practice, you will condition your arms for pom routine performance. **Emphasize the triceps as they are often weaker than the biceps** and they are important in all pushing motions.

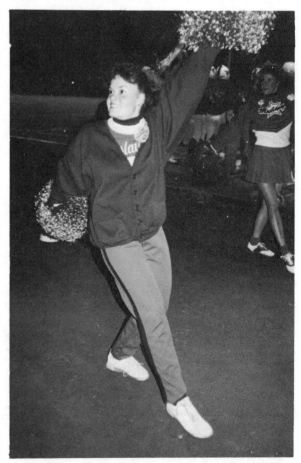

Figure 11-12

> *"Our dance routines consist of lots of back arches. Is there any special way to condition to increase the arch in my back?"*

BACK

A back arch can be performed by beginning in a standing position, then lifting your chest to the ceiling, hyperextending your back and following with your head. Since the **abdominals support the pelvis and are a major factor in aligning the lower back,** it makes sense to keep them at high levels of strength. In fact, all muscle groups involved in the lower back should be stretched and strengthened in a balanced way. Of course **any hyperextension of the spine should be executed with caution.** Try to "feel" yourself lifting up instead of back. Using the hinge method (a lean backward with a straight back, knees bent and on toes) of a back release instead of a complete arch is preferred technique to properly support the back. Remember, never completely release your neck in an arch! (Fig. 11-13) Instead, tilt your head back by lifting your chin to the ceiling. Assuming that you have no sign of individual posture problems you should be able to develop back arch capabilities by stretching the muscles in the front of your upper body and strengthening those in back.

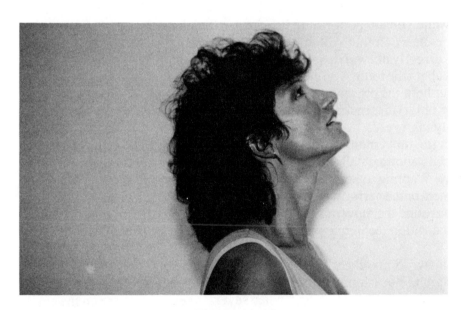

Use caution on head rolls; never throw head back; instead, lift chin up.

Figure 11-13

> *"I feel so clumsy when I dance and I know my facial projection is poor. What can I do to help get over this?"*

PROJECTING AND PERFORMING

Dance develops what it demands. If you train with low attention or energy, you will get limited development. **Your best aid to learning is not a teacher, but a good sense of humor.** Don't be afraid to make mistakes. Mistakes are necessary for learning. Enjoyment is an important part of training. Your performing strategy should involve the right mental, emotional and physical approach to the whole performance. This means radiating a positive, relaxed, confident attitude, no matter what insecurities or doubts may bubble up in your mind. Just pay attention to remaining relaxed, and keeping a bright, lively and alert expression on your face.

Dancing is an expression and communication of the body. Try to visualize yourself as part of the music and create an image, story, or character in your mind and your body will follow. **Using the face and a focus contributes to a more expressive performance** and as with all other aspects of the performance, this, too, must be practiced. It is never too early to remind yourself to direct focus out instead of down.

If you tell yourself to smile while you are performing it seems artificial, doesn't it? Instead, try to develop a relaxed and pleasant expression that will enhance your performance more than a routine filled with forced smiles. **Focus directly outward;** actually see something and relate to it visually. By making eye contact with objects about the room, you can present a more confident and direct approach, reflecting a sense of control over both the presentation and the routine. This sense of control is then automatically transmitted to the observers, making them more comfortable. As a result, the overall performance can be dramatically improved.

If you can find enjoyment in the movement, to experience it rather than simply go through it and to perform for pleasure, this will auotmatically be reflected in your face. Performers are often inconsistent in their presentation. Wanting to be received well, they try to perform for everyone else, never really enjoying the movement or the performance themselves. If you perform it for yourself first, thoroughly enjoying the experience and the movements, the audience will find it far more pleasurable. Refer to the relaxation and visualization techniques explained in chapter six.

Finally, there is that **"extra magic."** Some cheerleaders have it, others do not . . . it is psychic energy and like any energy, it is an intangible. You cannot see or feel it though the results are visually apparent during performance. The magic of this energy can be seen when several cheerleaders are on the court, all dancing the same movements in the same manner, yet one individual seems to stand out above the others. Your eyes seem to be continually drawn to the one with the extra something . . . that magic quality. It can be felt in the form of a kind of electricity which connects that performer to each individual in the audience. It is up to you to identify and tap that energy within. It is there for you to use and it will make the difference between mechanically going through the movements, or giving life and vitality to the performance. Remember, dancing is a part of you, so be yourself!

EVALUATING YOUR PROGRESS
Chapter Twelve

WHY EVALUATE?

No one wants to waste time, and that is exactly what happens if your conditioning efforts are not giving you the results you want. This is the key reason for testing. Periodic checks help you in three ways:
1. Keep your workouts efficient and effective
2. Keep you motivated
3. Help prevent injuries

EFFICIENT WORKOUTS

First and foremost, **applying your fitness testing results is vital for keeping your workout program as efficient and effective as possible.** Testing helps you **make sure** the exercises you are doing are helping you get the most benefits for your efforts. Based on the results of your fitness checks, you can make adjustments in the frequency, intensity, or duration of your exercise program. You will also be able to apply the principles of "overload" and "progressive resistance" (see chapter 2 and 4) which are key factors in helping you reach your peak athletic performance.

MOTIVATION

One of the best motivators for conditioning is finding out your actual progress! Both the positive and negative results of testing will help inspire you to train with greater intensity. The achievement of fitness and specific skills goals is possibly the greatest motivating force behind the mental discipline and physical effort necessary for a quality conditioning program.

INJURY PREVENTION

The final role of evaluation in the process of conditioning is preventative in nature. The careful screening and evaluation of daily workout records and fitness testing results is the simplest and most effective method for preventing the symptoms of overtraining (see chapter 4), such as fatigue, overuse injuries, and declining skill execution.

WHEN TO EVALUATE
ACUTE EVALUATION

The first type of testing frequency is called **acute evaluation.** These evaluations are done often — daily, weekly or at least twice a month. Your coach or captain can easily perform acute testing by analyzing your skills and/or workouts. You will focus on the following:
1. The general quality of your workout.
2. The specific ability to complete the prescribed number of sets and reps.
3. The effect conditioning has on performing specific skills.

CHRONIC EVALUATION

Chronic evaluation is different from acute testing. It is more elaborate involving measurements in all areas of fitness and it requires hours or days to complete. Chronic testing is performed at regularly scheduled intervals throughout the year, for example, pre, mid and post-season or annual/bi-annual. A coach or physical trainer should perform this type of testing.

PRINCIPLES OF FITNESS TESTING

SPECIFICITY

Before we learn how to test, we need to understand the general principles about testing. The most important factor that will make your fitness evaluation accurate and meaningful is applying the principle of specificity to your testing. **This means to test for what you are training!** Conditioning programs produce gains in fitness specific to the area of your body which is being overloaded. This idea is involved when you test a particular area of fitness (flexibility, strength, power, endurance, etc.). For example, if you are training to increase your power, it doesn't make much sense to have your muscular endurance tested.

GOALS

You and your squad must set specific goals for improvement, otherwise, your progress checks won't mean anything! After you set your goals, you must determine the specific characteristics of fitness that affect your performance of a skill. You will then test each of these areas that affect the skill(s) you are trying to master. If you are testing your general fitness, you must determine the importance of each test based on how that area of fitness relates to your goals. For example, you goal is to improve the power and height of your jumps. Your test should focus on your height increase and your lower body strength. Evaluations should have weighted scored assigned to each test which will reflect the importance of each area to your goal accomplishment.

RECORD KEEPING

Keep accurate records and keep it fun! Try setting up inner-squad competitions for reaching individual goals. Individual files can be maintained for each cheerleader as well as for the squad. It is very important to check your progress based on **your starting point;** use team averages and normal standards only as a guideline for comparison. Squad files can show team averages, the percent of increases or decreases in strength, power, endurance, and additional goal oriented records.

HOW TO EVALUATE

There are several ways to determine fitness including in-depth testing by trainers/sports physicians and simple tests that can be handled by fellow squad members or your coach. Both methods have been presented in this chapter. How you select a test will depend upon several factors, including: availability of equipment and personnel to administer testing, time required to obtain final results, cost of measurement, needs of program, etc.

The following paragraphs describe fitness evaluation for the major areas of fitness, proceeding from simple field measurements to some of the more advanced laboratory techniques which have been developed in the disciplines of exercise physiology and biomechanics. The easier tests can be handled by your coach; several others require an experience trainer, physical therapist or sports doctor to administer. Some squads won't have the advantage of having a trainer or doctor who can perform the more advanced testing . . . but do check around . . . you never know until you ask!

QUANTITATIVE VERSUS QUALITATIVE TESTING

Throughout the explanations we will discuss **qualitative versus qualitative measurements.** Qualitative simply means subjective testing and is the easier (but less accurate) of the two. Quantitative means **numerical or objective** testing. A sample evaluation chart (Table 12-9) is provided at the end of this chapter to help you start your own fitness testing.

FLEXIBILITY
DYNAMIC PERFORMANCE TESTING (coach/squad)

Possibly the easiest and most direct measurements of flexibility involve tests of dynamic performance or the **evaluation of a fitness area as it relates to the execution of a particular cheerleading skill.** Captains or coaches can definitely handle this type of testing. These tests determine the range of motion about a particular joint by 1) observing whether or not a given position can be obtained or 2) by evaluating a specific skill. Examples include splits, jumps and gymnastics skills. Since hamstring, quadricep and hip abductor/adductor flexibility is associated with the performance of many cheerleading skills, you can evaluate the degree of split in all three directions (right, left and front) to get an indication of your current degree of flexibility in these muscle groups.

RANGE OF MOTION (ROM) TESTING (administer by a trainer or physician)

Although tests of dynamic performance are adequate to know qualitative information, to actually measure the range of motion about a joint or changes in a joint's flexibility, we need to use a slightly more sophisticated approach. A measurement device called a goniometer can be used to determine the degree of flexibility in a given joint. A **goniometer** can be used to measure virtually all joints in their various directions of movement (Fig. 12-2) by placing the center of the instrument at the fulcrum of the joint and aligning the arms with he longitudinal axis of each moving body segment. Accurate measurements require that specific anatomical landmarks be used as reference points and that repeated measurements be taken by the same individual. Be sure to allow cheerleaders to warm up adequately before beginning the test.

LOWER BACK, HIP, AND HAMSTRING TESTING (administer by coach or trainer)

The **sit and reach test** (Fig. 12-3a and 12-3b) is designed to evaluate the flexibility of the lower back,

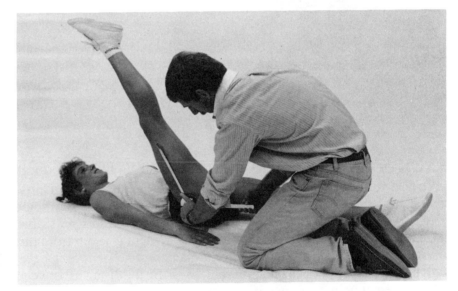

Figure 12-2: (Goniometry) Range of Motion-Hip Flexion

hamstrings and hips. To perform the test have the cheerleader sit with legs extended fully. The feet are placed flat against the box* with arms extended and the index fingers of both hands together. Have the cheerleader stretch forward as far as possible and note the distance reached. Repeat the test twice more and take the best score. (*A yardstick should be attached to the top of the box with a fourteen-inch mark placed at the point where the feet contact the box.)

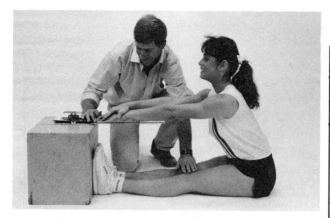

Figure 12-3A

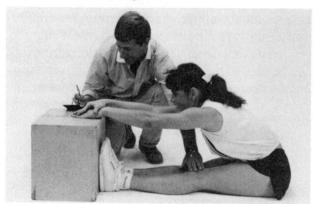

Figure 12-3B

Table 12.1.	SIT & REACH TEST	
Sit and reach score	**Fitness level**	
11 in or less	Very poor	_____
12 to 13 in	Poor	_____
14 to 16 in	Average	_____
16 to 18 in	Good	_____
20 to 21 in	Very good	_____
22 to 23 in	Excellent	_____
24+ in	Superior	_____

BACK HYPERTENSION FLEXIBILITY TEST (coach or trainer)

To determine the range of lower back extension, the **back hypertension test** (Fig. 12-4a and 12-4b) can be performed. Have the cheerleader lie down in a prone position on the floor, with the feet held in place. With hands placed behind the head the cheerleader will slowly and gently lift the chin and chest as far off the floor as possible. A measurement is taken from the floor to the sternal notch (the groove at the top of the sternum where the clavicle attaches). Next, have the cheerleader sit on the floor with the back and buttocks against a wall. Measure the distance between the floor and the sternal notch (seated sternal height). Lower back flexibility is determined by the following equation:

$$\text{Back hypertension} = \frac{\text{Hyperextension height} \times 10}{\text{(seated sternal height)}}$$

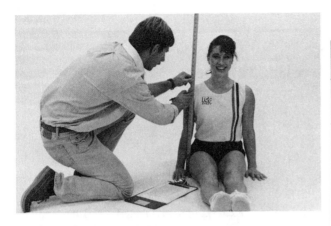

Figure 12-4A

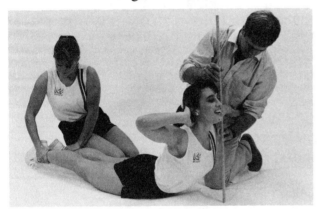

Figure 12-4B

Table 12.2.	Back Hyperextension Test	
Flexibility score	**Fitness level**	
25 or lower	Very poor	_____
26-35	Poor	_____
36-45	Average	_____
46-50	Good	_____
51-55	Very good	_____
56-57	Excellent	_____
58+	Superior	_____

CARDIORESPIRATORY ENDURANCE

OBSERVANCE TESTS AND HEART RATE MONITORING

As with flexibility, **tests of performance** can be used to qualitatively determine cardiorespiratory endurance. This is done by observing your ability to complete the required workout or performance without getting overly fatigued. You can simply observe the obvious signs of fatigue or monitor your heart rate for a more specific measurement of your endurance level. Chapter 3 gives a complete explanation how to check your heart rate following aerobic exercise.

12 MINUTE RUN (coach/squad)

An easy to administer quantitative field test, called the **12 minute run,** has been shown to correlate well with laboratory determinations of cardiorespiratory endurance. The only tools required are a measured track (preferably 1/4 mile in length) and a stop watch. The test begins by having cheerleaders warm up properly and remove their watches. Following the start command, cheerleaders run continuously for 12 minutes. The object is to run the greatest distance possible at a pace which can be consistently maintained for 12 minutes. The removal of watches prior to the test is a deterrent to pushing harder near the end of the run in order to gain additional distance. The final distance achieved is measured to the closest 1/4 mile and compared against norms, a particular goal or a previous score (Table 12-3).

Table 12-3.   **12-MINUTE WALKING/RUNNING TEST**
Distance (Miles) Covered in 12 Minutes

Fitness Category			13-19	20-29	Age (Years) 30-39	40-49	50-59	60+
I.	Very Poor	(men)	<1.30*	<1.22	<1.18	<1.14	<1.03	<.87
		(women)	<1.0	<.96	<.94	<.88	<.84	<.78
II.	Poor	(men)	1.30-1.37	1.22-1.31	1.18-1.30	1.14-1.24	1.03-1.16	.87-1.02
		(women)	1.00-1.18	.96-1.11	.95-1.05	.88- .98	.84- .93	.78- .86
III.	Fair	(men)	1.38-1.56	1.32-1.49	1.31-1.45	1.25-1.39	1.17-1.30	1.03-1.20
		(women)	1.19-1.29	1.12-1.22	1.06-1.18	.99-1.11	.94-1.05	.87- .98
IV.	Good	(men)	1.57-1.72	1.50-1.64	1.46-1.56	1.40-1.53	1.31-1.44	1.21-1.32
		(women)	1.30-1.43	1.23-1.34	1.19-1.29	1.12-1.24	1.06-1.18	.99-1.09
V.	Excellent	(men)	1.73-1.86	1.65-1.76	1.57-1.69	1.54-1.65	1.45-1.58	1.33-1.55
		(women)	1.44-1.51	1.35-1.45	1.30-1.39	1.25-1.34	1.19-1.30	1.10-1.18
VI.	Superior	(men)	>1.87	>1.77	>1.70	>1.66	>1.59	>1.56
		(women)	>1.52	>1.46	>1.40	>1.35	>1.31	>1.19

*< Means "less than"; > means "more than."

1.5-MILE RUN TEST
Time (Minutes)

Fitness Category			13-19	20-29	Age (Years) 30-39	40-49	50-59	60+
I.	Very Poor	(men)	>15:31*	>16:01	>16:31	>17:31	>19:01	>2:01
		(women)	>18:31	>19:01	>19:31	>20:01	>20:31	>21:01
II.	Poor	(men)	12:11-15:30	14:01-16:00	14:44-16:30	15:36-17:30	17:01-19:00	19:01-20:00
		(women)	18:30-16:55	19:00-18:31	19:30-19:01	20:00-19:31	20:30-20:01	21:00-21:31
III.	Fair	(men)	10:49-12:10	12:01-14:00	12:31-14:45	13:01-15:35	14:31-17:00	16:16-19:00
		(women)	16:54-14:31	18:30-15:55	19:00-16:31	19:30-17:31	20:00-19:01	20:30-19:31
IV.	Good	(men)	9:41-10:48	10:46-12:00	11:01-12:30	11:31-13:00	12:31-14:30	14:00-16:15
		(women)	14:30-12:30	15:54-13:31	16:30-14:31	17:30-15:56	19:00-16:31	19:30-17:31
V.	Excellent	(men)	8:37- 9:40	9:45-10:45	10:00-11:00	10:30-11:30	11:00-12:30	11:15-13:59
		(women)	12:29-11:50	13:30-12:30	14:30-13:00	15:55-13:45	16:30-14:30	17:30-16:30
VI.	Superior	(men)	< 8:37	< 9:45	<10:00	<10:30	<11:00	<11:15
		(women)	<11:50	<12:30	<13:00	<13:45	<14:30	<16:30

*< Means "less than"; > means "more than."

MAXIMAL OXYGEN CONSUMPTION (trainer/physician)

Another test of cardiorespiratory endurance is performed in a laboratory setting where a cheerleader runs or cycles to exhaustion. The total volume of air expired per minute is measured and collected gas samples are analyzed for oxygen and carbon dioxide concentrations. These values are then used to calculate the **maximal oxygen consumption or VO 2 max.** When available, this test provides the best indicate of general cardiorespiratory fitness; however, the information obtained is specific to the activity performed and may not correlate well with endurance in other forms of aerobic activity. In other words, a laboratory test of a cheerleader's cardiorespiratory fitness with regards to running or cycling may not give us a quantitative indication of their endurance specific to cheerleading.

Table 12-4.			FITNESS LEVEL				
Age (years)	Very poor	Poor	Average	Good	Very good	Excellent	Superior
Males							
17-29	0-17	17-35	36-41	42-47	48-50	51-55	55+
30-39*	0-13	13-26	27-32	33-38	39-43	44-48	48+
40-49	0-11	11-22	23-27	28-33	34-38	39-43	43+
50-59	0-8	8-16	17-21	22-28	29-33	34-38	38+
60-69	0-6	6-12	13-17	18-24	25-30	31-35	35+
Females							
17-29	0-14	14-28	29-32	33-35	36-42	43-47	47+
30-39*	0-11	11-22	23-28	29-34	35-40	41-45	45+
40-49	0-9	9-18	19-23	24-30	31-34	35-40	40+
50-59	0-6	6-12	13-17	18-24	25-30	31-35	35+
60-69	0-5	5-10	11-14	15-20	21-25	26-30	30+

MUSCULAR ENDURANCE
STATIC ENDURANCE (ISOMETRIC CONTRACTION) (coach/trainer)

Quantification of muscular endurance, both static and dynamic, can be determined by using **calibrated weights** and **specific exercises.** One method to determine if an athlete has adequate muscular endurance is through a test of static endurance (i.e. isometric contraction) meaning the measurement of the maximal time a cheerleader can hold a specified weight in a given position. An example would be the length of time a base could support a mounter's weight in an overhead press.

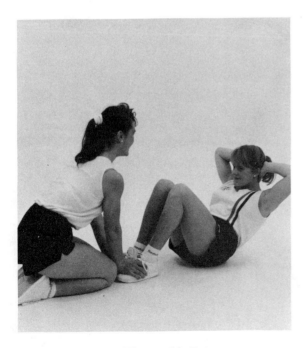

Figure 12-5

DYNAMIC ENDURANCE (CONCENTRIC AND ECCENTRIC CONTRACTION) (coach/squad)

Dynamic endurance can be tested by the number of reps over a given time period or the number of reps at a given weight. Examples of repetitions over a given time period would be the number of sit ups performed in one minute (Fig. 12-5) or the number of consecutive jumps or kicks that can be performed in a time limit. Examples of testing the maximum number of repetitions at a given weight could be simply the number of jumps a cheerleader can perform or the number of bench presses at 75 percent of body weight.

STRENGTH AND POWER

Measuring muscular strength is relatively simple and can be done by having a cheerleader perform a one repetition maximal lift (e.g. bench press or squat). However, as we have previously observed, most skills in cheerleading involve the generation of power. Although strength is inherent in the creation of power, **tests of strength do not give us accurate information about a cheerleader's ability to generate power.** In fact, at present there are few simple tests of power which can be performed without sophisticated laboratory equipment such as isokinetic exercise machines (Fig. 12-6).

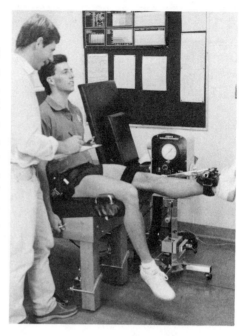

Figure 12-6

VERTICAL JUMP AND OLYMPIC LIFTS (squad/coach/trainer)

Of the field methods currently in used the **best indicators of lower body power generation** are tests of **vertical jump** and the weight used in a one repetition maximum for the **Olympic lifts** (clean, jerk and snatch). The vertical jump test is administered by first recording the cheerleader's initial extended arm height. This is followed by having the cheerleader take a deep squat (no preparatory steps allowed) (Fig. 12-7a) and jump to touch the maximal height on the wall (Fig. 12-7b). Measure the difference between the two heights and record the best jump in three trials (Table 12-5). This technique can be modified for use in determining jump "prep" height and the maximal height produced in "toss or pop" stunt preps (Fig. 12-7c).

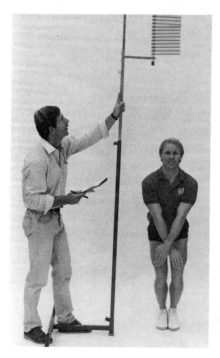

Figure 12-7A

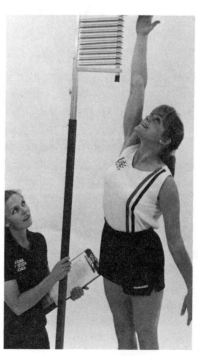

Figure 12-7B

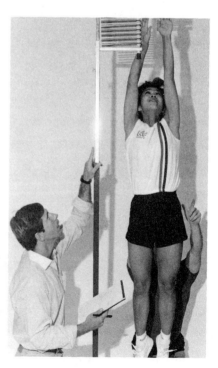

Figure 12-7C

Table 12-5.	LEG POWER SCORE	
Difference between prejump and postjump touch marks	**Fitness Level**	
7 in	Very poor	_____
10 in	Poor	_____
16 in	Average	_____
18 in	Good	_____
20 in	Very Good	_____
22 in	Excellent	_____
24+ in	Superior	_____

NUTRITION

Unfortunately, people usually don't check nutritional habits until a problem exists. And even the absence of symptoms is not adequate evidence to support the claim that we have a nutritionally sound diet! Consider nutrition as the missing clue to peak performance, you know, that extra special advantage for a top athlete. Most advanced athletes (for instance, people training to be in the Olympics) understand the **vital effect nutritional health has on performance and overall fitness.** But how many cheerleaders do you know that choose the apple instead of the french fries? And usually the only worry about the french fries is calories, not the effect they have on your ability to perform!

The easiest way to check your nutritional health is to keep a list (Table 12-6) of the foods you eat over several days and evaluate it. Check for caloric content, vitamin and mineral content and the percentage of calories from fats (saturated or unsaturated), proteins (essential and nonessential) and carbohydrates (single versus complex). (See chapter 7.) In addition, a **consultation from a registered dietician (R.D.) or a nutritionist** is a great way to get practical information on nutrition.

Table 12-6.	ONE WEEK NUTRITION DIETARY DIARY		
Date	**Meal**	**Food/Beverage**	**Quantity**
_____	_____	_____	_____
_____	_____	_____	_____
_____	_____	_____	_____

BODY COMPOSITION

Visual inspection and the way in which your clothes fit can be used to qualitatively (subjectively) evaluate changes in your body composition. However, even experts can be deceived! The actual measurement of body composition generally requires the use of laboratory equipment ranging from simple calipers to complex instrumentation which determines the presence of radioactive potassium. Of the many techniques which exist, there are two which provide relatively accurate information at a reasonable expense of time and money.

SKINFOLD MEASUREMENT (trainer/physician)

The determination of body composition by **skinfold thickness measurement** involves the use of calipers placed at specific places on the body. This measurement gives an estimate of the subcutaneous (below the skin) fat which is then used in population specific (i.e. groups matched for age, sex, etc.) equations for the calculation of percent body fat. This method requires training and practice in identifying the sites for caliper placement and caliper use. In addition, the appropriate equation must be selected specific to the age and sex of the cheerleader.

The body composition of young adult women is estimated from the thickness of the tricep (Fig. 12-8a) and suprailiac (Fig. 12-8a) skinfolds, while the amount of subcutaneous fat at the subscapular (Fig. 12-8c) and thigh (Fig. 12-8d) sites are used for young adult men. These formulas have since been converted into nomograms for a simplified method of estimating percent body fat (Tables 12-7a and 12-7b.) The technique for measuring skinfolds follows.

SKINFOLD MEASUREMENT TECHNIQUE

1. Measure all skinfolds on the same side of the body, using calipers which exert ten grams per square millimeter on the caliper face.
2. Grasp the skinfold firmly between the thumb and forefinger, making sure to include two layers of skin and subcutaneous fat, without the underlying muscle.
3. Apply the caliper one centimeter below the fingers, to a depth equal to the width of the skinfold being measured.
4. Measure the thickness along the natural fold of the skin (i.e. vertical for triceps and thigh, diagonal for suprailiac and subscapular).
5. Measurements are completed for all sites and then repeated. If a difference of greater than 0.05 millimeters exists, a third measurement is required. Use the mean of the two closest values to represent the skinfold thickness for a particular site.
6. Skinfold sites are as follows:

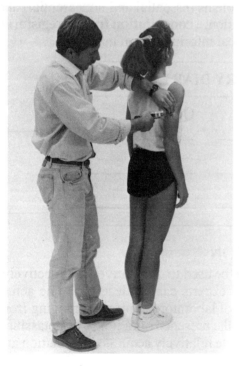

Figure 12-8A

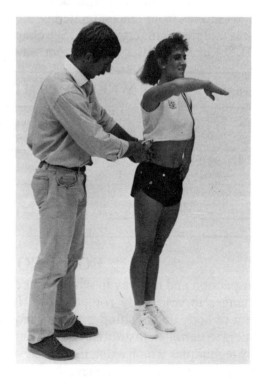

Figure 12-8A

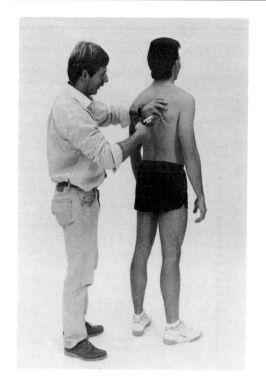

Figure 12-8C

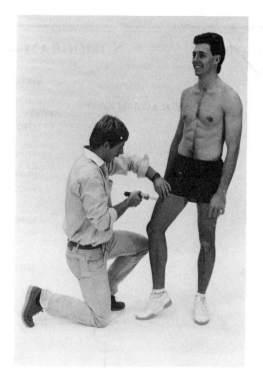

Figure 12-8D

Table 12-7A   **NOMOGRAM — YOUNG MEN**

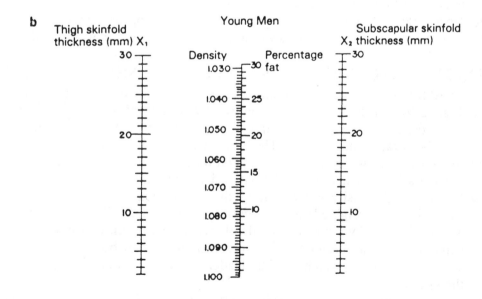

Table 12-7B   NOMOGRAM — YOUNG WOMEN

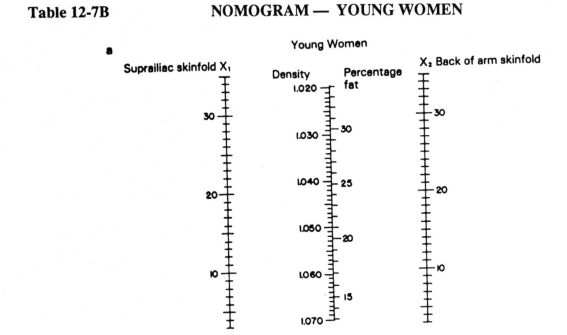

(Percent body fat and body density are determined by drawing a straight line joining the two skinfold values and noting the values at which it intersects the middle column.)

Although the basic techniques of measurement are relatively simple, even highly trained individuals can expect **5-7 percent error in the final calculated percent body fat.** This error is due to fluctuations in body water, inaccurate or inconsistent caliper site selection, improper caliper use, selection of inappropriate conversion equation, as well as variation inherent in the use of standardized equations.

HYDROSTATIC DETERMINATION OF BODY DENSITY (trainer/physician)

The best standard for the measurement of body composition is the **hydrostatic determination of body density** (Fig. 12-9). This technique, commonly called **underwater weighing,** involves a series of measurements whose results are converted into an estimation of body density which is then used to calculate percent body fat via an equation. The basic idea is that lean tissue (muscle, organs, bone, etc.) has a greater density than water (i.e. it will float on water). A cheerleader with a high percentage of body fat will have a low density and will float easily when put into water. Conversely, a lean cheerleader will have a high density and will find it difficult to float when placed in water.

The cheerleader is initially weighted on a conventional scale, followed by either the estimation or actual determination of residual volume. Residual volume is the **amount of air** which remains in the lungs following maximal expiration and therefore its contribution to the body buoyancy must be taken into account. Several trials, during which the cheerleader is weighed underwater in a chair attached to a balance, are then performed.

Prior to submersion the cheerleader must exhale fully to remove the buoyancy associated with this volume of air. The accuracy of this technique depends on many factors including: accurate determination of residential volume, the sensitivity of scales and the ability of the cheerleader to remain motionless in the chair following full expiration of the lung's volume. The most errors are found when using a standard equation which converts the results of the underwater weights to a body density. This is due to the incorrect assumption that all lean tissue has the same relative density. However, even in the face of all these potential sources of error, **the accuracy for this method of determining body composition is generally within 3 percent.**

Table 12-9.	Percent Body Fat Norms:	
	Female	**Male**
Athletic	15%	10%
Average	20%	15%
Obese	30%	25%

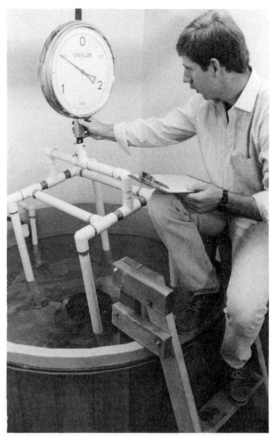

Figure 12-9

PSYCHOLOGICAL

The evaluation of psychological skills and mental status as it relates to cheerleading performance has been described in detail in chapter 7. That information will not be presented again here. Just remember: Your mental abilities to visualize, concentrate, relax and remain calm affect your performance as much or more than any physical ability. Make sure your squad understands the importance of good psychological skills.

In summary, remember testing will keep your workout program efficient and effective, motivating, and help prevent injuries. As you set your goals, consider the principles of specificity and keep good records. Perform simple progress checks as often as you can and set up in-depth testing one to three times per year. Check flexibility, strength, power, and endurance. Don't forget that nutrition and body composition also affect your performance. Most of all, keep it fun and keep it challenging! After all, that's what being an athlete is all about!

Table 12-10.

SAMPLE EVALUATION PROGRAM

Name: _____

Date: _____

Area of Fitness	**Test**		**Score**	**%Change**
Flexibility	Split:	front ___	yes/no	
		right ___	yes/no	
		left ___	yes/no	
	Sit and reach		inches	
	Back hypertension		percent	
	Shoulder goniom.		degrees	
Endurance				
Cardiorespiratory	12 min. run		miles	
Muscular	Sit ups		# and minutes	
	B52's medicine ball		# and minutes	
	Dips		maximum #	
	Chin ups		maximum #	
Strength/power	Vertical jump		inches	
	Stunt prep height		inches	
	Overhead press		pounds	
	Clean/jerk		pounds	
Body Composition	Skin-fold test			
	with calipers			

INJURY PREVENTION
Chapter Thirteen

Cheerleaders are highly specialized athletes. Along with the specific activities associated with cheerleading comes the potential for injuries which may or may not be limited to cheerleading, but are associated with virtually all specialized athletes. In treating cheerleading injuries for sixteen years, injuries have remained fairly constant. Seventy-four percent of cheerleading injuries are simply strains, sprains and contusions; and these injuries are no more frequent today than in earlier years! With over 600,000 participants, cheerleading is one of the most important and beneficial activities in our school system, and through education, training and supervision we can all do our part in keeping the activity as safe as possible!

HOW MANY INJURIES OCCUR?

Statistics show that cheerleading is quite a safe activity. Compared to most other athletic activities, cheerleaders experience an incredibly low rate of injuries. One survey reported in 1986 there were 600,000* participants in cheerleading compared to 441,000* participants in girls basketball. Reported injuries for cheerleading were only 6,911 (1 percent) compared to 101,000 (23 percent) reported for girls basketball. Thirteen percent or 13,000 girls basketball participants received injuries severe enough to be out for the entire season; this is twice the number of total cheerleading injuries.

Let's look at high school football for the same year. In 1986 there were 1,048,100 high school football participants and 636,279 injuries; in other words, 61 percent of football players received injuries. Sixteen and one-half percent of the injuries were moderate (out 8-21 days); 86 percent kept participants out more than 21 days; 25 percent of the injuries due to football keep participants out for more than 21 days.

WHERE TO BEGIN

Injuries that occur in cheerleading run the gamut from a dislocated finger to a compression fracture of the lumbar spine. To address all of these would take volumes and could not be adequately covered in this short discourse. However, we will attempt to outline some of the reasons injuries occur, discuss how to help prevent them and give you some general rules for treatment of common injuries which occur in cheerleading. The following specific examples are designed to provoke discussions that will help you realize some of the problem areas with regard to cheerleading injuries. In addition, you will learn how to recognize and respond to those problems in a professional and confident manner.

TERMINOLOGY

Let's start by defining some commonly used terms that we encounter in the athletic injury field. These terms will help us be at the same level as far as talking about specific injuries, their prevention and treatment. This is by no means a complete list, rather a starting point.

• **Ligament** — A band or sheet of strong fibrous connective tissue, connecting the articular end of bones (the ends that move) serving to bind them together so as to facilitate or limit movement.

• **Tendon** — Fibrous connective tissue serving as the attachment of muscles to bones or other anatomical structures.

• **Sprain** — Injury to a ligament which is measured by degrees: 1st degree = minimal damage and stretching; 2nd degree = severe stretching or partial tear; 3rd degree = tearing or complete disruption of an attachment of the tissue itself.

• **Strain** — Injury involving the muscle, tendon or musculotendenous unit which, as with a sprain, is classified by degrees.

• **Chondromalacia** — The softening or destruction of articular cartilage often seen at the knee joint.

- **Bursa** — A sac-like cavity that allows the muscle or tendon to slide over bone.
- **Meniscus** — Intra-articular fibrocatilage of crescent shape found in certain joints, especially the lateral and medial cartilage of the knee joint.
- **Subluxation** — Incomplete or partial dislocation of a joint.
- **Dislocation** — The displacement of a bone from its normal position in a joint.
- **Acute** — Having rapid onset. Severe symptoms in a short course. Not chronic.
- **Chronic** — Long, drawn out. Applies to a disease or injury that is not acute.
- **Heat Exhaustion** — An acute reaction to heat exposure with weakness, dizziness, nausea, headaches and collapse. Skin cold and clammy, pupils dilated.
- **Heat Stroke** (hyperpyrexia) — A dangerous reaction to heat exposure with high body temperature, cessation of sweating, headaches, numbness, confusion, fast pulse and possible delirium.

PRIMARY ELEMENTS OF INJURY

LACK OF CONDITIONING

Although a large number of cheerleading injuries happen by accident, there are some significant problematic areas to be addressed that can dramatically decrease the chances of an accident happening. A primary area is the **lack of conditioning** for a particular activity or stunt. For example, if partner stunts require work above the head, it is imperative that the bases of these stunts have strong upper bodies, particularly in the area of the cervical spine (neck) and upper trapezius musculature (shoulders). Care needs to be taken to strengthen these areas, throughout a joint's full range of motion. Tight muscles or joint capsules lead to unnecessary stress forces on ligaments, tendons and the surrounding musculature. These stresses cause the supporting tissue to be stretched or even tear, leading to an injury which manifests itself as swelling, tenderness and discoloration of the affected area.

In addition to inadequate strength and flexibility, lack of proper conditioning also lends itself to injuries toward the end of practices or games as athletes become tired, they are more susceptible to being hurt. Cheerleaders are no exception. Remember that **fatigue** is sometimes not judged well by participants themselves but better by the sponsor/coach or even the other squad members. Be aware of times when your muscles are too fatigued to do a stunt or tumble correctly. If your muscles and joints are tired, don't ask them to do something they can't accomplish. Muscles that don't work, shouldn't! Rest, fluid replacement and time are necessary to enable the muscles and joints to recover properly.

IMPROPER ENVIRONMENT

Another factor that enters into the injury pattern is the **improper environment.** As we know, not all game situation environments are perfect, but practice environments should be close. Cinder tracks, hardwood floors and wet grass need to be as safe as possible with regard to slips and falls. Crash mats and spotters, as well as caution, are excellent ways of improving the environment in which you practice to make the stunts and pyramids safer. Spotters are recommended when learning stunts, tumbling and pyramids and when performing many difficult skills. Never perform any skill until it has been mastered completely during practice. Wiping shoes off before stunts and making sure there are no wet spots on the floor or grass are necessary measures to insure the safety of the squad. These things seem small and unimportant but they can make the difference between being safe or being injured. An excellent way to prepare for particular adverse environments is to practice ways to make them safe and work out under those improved conditions. If a particular stadium or gym has a poor environment for cheerleading, scout it out and find ways to improve that environment. In the instance that the environment can't be improved, decide which skills should not be used because of the unsafe conditions. It seems like a lot of work, but it will pay off in a safer performance, with less chance of injuries.

IMPROPER TRAINING

Injuries go hand in hand with **improper training.** If stunts are not practiced correctly and mastered, they should never be done in a competition or game situation. Even the most basic stunts can go awry and lead to a severe injury. Specific stunts require specific muscle groups that need to be strengthened. If they are not strong enough then don't attempt the stunts. It's not worth the risk. A major component of proper training is general stretching prior to each practice or each game (see chapter 5). This is sometimes boring and tedious, but it serves an important function. It allows the muscles, tendons and ligaments time to warm up gradually and be stretched gently without any abnormal forces applied to them. It also allows for the vascular system (blood supply) to increase its flow to the musculature and connective tissue associated with the particular activity or stunt. This is the true meaning of warming up. This helps prevent any sudden stretching forces on the joints which are normally the culprits in strains, sprains and dislocations. Training for cheerleading as with any other sport requires a strict commitment. A commitment to a safe, injury-free year for you and your squad requires many hours of workout and practice.

TREATMENT AND REHABILITATION
WHAT TO DO IF AN INJURY OCCURS

Strength training and flexibility exercises are imperative if you are to be at your best, which is also the most efficient way to prevent a season-ending injury. However, even though you take all the precautions we have mentioned above, there is still the possibility of injury. The next major question that arises is, "What to do if an injury occurs?" **Make sure your coach understands basic first-aid techniques so that injuries will be taken seriously.** For discussion purposes, let's examine a sprain of the ankle, as it is a fairly common injury which is relatively simple to handle. As we all have seen or experienced personally, the ankle is generally injured by a sudden inversion (inward twisting motion). This commonly happens on an uneven surface when dismounting from a stunt, jumping or finishing a tumbling pass. Speaking in medical terms, the lateral ligaments of the ankle, the anterior talofibular ligament, the calcaneofibular ligament and the posterior talofibular ligament are compromised. There may be effusion in the joint capsule, discoloration and pain along with noticeable swelling and point tenderness just inferior to the lateral malleoli. Suffice it to say, it is a touch more complicated than the definition we used earlier, but in fact this is the symptomatology we see time after time. It is important to remember that although it is obviously not a life-threatening injury, it may be much more severe than most people tend to treat it. There are a number of concerns that must be addressed, including the possibility of a small fracture in the medial portion of the dome of the talus. This presents itself as the ankle sprain that won't get well, or "just gives way." There is also tenderness with passive plantar flexion (pointing the toe), as well as pain inferior to the medial malleoli (inside ankle bone). But enough on this tangent and back to our simple ankle sprain.

THE "R.I.C.E." RULE OF THUMB

Remember the rule of thumb for the treatment of sprains and strains is to use **rest, ice, compression and elevation** (which conveniently spells "R I C E"). All are important in the acute treatment of this injury. We can also see how they are used throughout the course of treatment and rehabilitation. Let's say our discussion injury is fairly severe with swelling, discoloration, tenderness and pain. In this case, as in all others, **don't play doctor.** It's not your job and it's doubtful you want the responsibility. Immediately, elevate it above the heart level and seek trained medical help. it is best to go to an emergency room or an emergency satellite clinic for an x-ray, to confirm that no bones have been broken, as well as to insure that proper care and rehabilitation is initiated. In our ankle injury we find that a stress x-ray reveals a secondary strain, probably without any tearing. Ankle injuries respond well to protective function, compression, weight bearing to tolerance and gentle active and passive range of motion. **Find an athletic trainer, a physical therapist or sports medicine physician who deals with these injuries on a daily basis and seek their help.** They are well versed in the newest and most progressive modalities to treat sports injuries and they can start the appropriate rehabilitation program immediately. Such specialists, physical therapists or athletic trainers can give you daily treatment that is consistent with the injury and rehabilitation program that will return you to action as soon as possible, with little or no danger of re-injury. They are often provided for high school and college athletes by school districts or universities. If they are not available, you can find a specialist in the phone book or through the local chapter of the American Medical Association.

Generally speaking, our discussion injury would respond well to daily treatment, for five to seven days with ice, intermittent compression, taping, high voltage stimulation, massage, gentle active and passive range of motion and weight bearing to tolerance with crutches. Following this period of time, full weight bearing should be pain free. Fast walking or slow straight line jogging would be started at this time, as well as strengthening exercises to recondition the musculature surrounding the ankle joint. Returning to practice on a limited basis would probably be permitted, provided tape was applied for support before working out and ice was applied after workout to prevent any further swelling or trauma to the joint. Treatment should be continued until normal activity without pain can be accomplished on a routine basis. Remember, give the injury time to heal. You are a part of a team, but working out half speed and with pain could be dangerous not only to you, but your partner or teammates as well. **Please understand that our discussion ankle is only an example and nothing will take the place of trained medical professional help when it comes to the diagnosis, care and rehabilitation of a specific injury.**

EMERGENCY CARE

Here are some general rules of thumb for commonly seen problems that are quite simple.

1. **If someone falls from a stunt or pyramid** and does not immediately get up, don't move them. Keep them still until trained help can get there. It may not be anything, but you are not trained, nor do you want to take that chance.
2. **If a joint "looks funny"** following a fall, don't try to fix it. You could cause more damage than the original problem.
3. **If you are not sure about something,** don't touch, don't move it and get trained medical help. There are too many specific situations to discuss here, as space will not permit it. These rules, as well as good common sense should help as an acceptable guide.

Please understand that we don't want to make you trainers, physical therapists or sports medicine physicians, but knowing what to do if an injury occurs can often times mean the difference between a good, speedy recovery and a poor one. Excellent references on general first aid can be obtained from your local Red Cross an emergency medical facility of from a variety of publications. One particularly good book with regards to sports injury and their rehabilitation is **SPORTS MEDICINE, PREVENTION EVALUATION MANAGEMENT AND REHABILITATION,** Stephen Roy and Richard Irvin, published by Prentice Hall, 1983. It is interesting reading and very understandable. It coves topics such as shoulders, wrists and hand injuries, groin pulls, back injuries and their care, hip pain, knee pain, shin splints, ankle problems, lacerations, turf burns and fractures.

COMMON QUESTIONS REGARDING CHEERLEADING INJURIES

"Our squad recently started requiring back hand springs for try outs, and now it seems that the majority of cheerleaders have wrist problems. What can be done to improve the situation?"

WRISTS

The possibility exists that there is an overuse syndrome developing in these wrists. Most probably, there has been repeated practice and secondary to this a stretching of the wrists flexors. There may also be some bruising of the carpal bones at the wrist joint. Prolonged rest would be excellent, but not practical in all situations. Therefore, protective taping or strapping will probably help with most of these problems, at least initially. A strengthening and flexibility program should be started to help the wrist joint become more stable and tolerate this activity better. A word of caution: if any swelling or severe pain occurs or if any numbness or tingling occurs in the hand or fingers, seek professional help. Wrists are very susceptible to these compression injuries and there are a great many nerves and tendons which pass across the wrist joint. There is also very little area for swelling to occur and if it does it puts pressure on these structures. This prolonged pressure can cause serious or even permanent damage.

> *"Virtually all co-ed partner stunts utilize a 'pop or toss' preparation which has led to some overused shoulders in the male cheerleaders on our squad. Is there any way to prevent these injuries without changing the basic stunt techniques?"*

SHOULDERS

Shoulder overuse is a catch-all term. You could be talking about a rotator cuff injury, subcromial bursitis, subdeltoid bursitis, bicipital tendonitis or rupture, acromioclavicular ligamentous injury or just plain weakness which leads to shoulder pain. Probably the culprit here is weakness of specific muscle structures in the shoulder complex. Strength training is the first area you should evaluate and it should begin very early in workouts. Strengthening the rotator cuff, the pectoralis musculature, the upper trapezius, all three portions of the deltoid muscle as well as the biceps and triceps, should help with the weakness and may even eliminate the pain. Nothing will substitute for genuine strength throughout the full range of motion when it comes to preventing injuries.

Shoulder injuries can be very complex, but shoulders that are strong and flexible are much less apt to be problematic or to develop an overuse syndrome.

> *"Personally I have had a bad lower back for several years and I would hate to have any of my cheerleaders have to suffer for the rest of their lives from a pyramid or stunt-induced strain. How can I help them reduce their changes of incurring a lifelong debilitating back injury?"*

BACK

Back injuries could comprise volumes of literature, and your question is an excellent one. Always remember the key terms: **stability, strength and flexibility.** A strong spine is a stable spine but it must be flexible also. Caution and exercise are the keys. There are a number of muscle groups that play a direct role in low back strength and flexibility. Obviously, the paraspinous muscles that run the length of the spine on either side just next to the center are very important. There are also some small muscles called the multifidus muscles that are extremely important in vertebral stability. They should be exercised routinely. A good exercise for both of these is to get on all fours and raise your right hand and your left leg at the same time, then switch sides, your left hand and your right leg. It looks funny but if you do this regularly it will help to strengthen and stabilize your back musculature. Remember to hold these on each side for a 3 to 4 count. Not as obviously, the hamstrings, gluteals, abdominals and the quadriceps also play a part in low back stability through the forces they impart on the pelvis and the trunk. Stabilized hamstring stretches, quadriceps stretching and strengthening and exercises to tighten the gluteal muscles are all important in low back stability and in preventing low back problems. A stretching and strengthening program can be done in 5 to 10 minutes along with your other warm-ups before practice or games. Done religiously it will decrease the chance of low back injuries and pain significantly.

> *"It never seems to fail. Each time we try and learn new stunts, either one of the partners or the spotter get hit in the face. Then we have someone with a shiner or a laceration that just keeps on bleeding."*

BRUISES AND CUTS

One positive thing about this is that you have a spotter to get hit! Shiners are just occupational hazards and they are hard to avoid. It may not seem so at the time but it's better to get a shiner than let your partner fall and sustain a worse injury. Caution needs to be used by both the spotter and the partners. Spotters should try to reach for the shoulders, chest or waist in a falling stunt and avoid using the head as a handle. It is hard to hold on to and it damages very easily. Facial lacerations that won't quit bleeding can be a problem. If, by chance, you have a hemophiliac or "free bleeder" on your squad, take the appropriate precautions to see that they don't get cut. Facial lacerations as a rule tend to look worse than they are. They bleed quite freely because of their rich vascularity or blood supply. All cuts should be kept as clean as possible. Ice and pressure to the area is imperative to help stop the blood and anesthetize the wound. Use a clean cloth or sterile compress if it's available. If the bleeding doesn't stop within 4 to 5 minutes or the cut looks fairly deep, get professional help. Facial or scalp lacerations need to be carefully sutured within the first few hours of the injury, not the next day. If you are not sure whether or not sutures are needed, then let a physician decide. It's better to be safe than sorry when it comes to a laceration of the face.

> *"I heard that someone having strong quadriceps could predispose cheerleaders to hamstring strains. I am not sure I understand how."*

HAMSTRING AND QUADRICEP

It would be difficult to say that strong quadriceps would predispose cheerleaders to have hamstring pulls. Physiologically, if the quads were extremely strong they could lengthen and there could be a possibility of a hamstring stretch or pull. This would not necessarily predispose a person to hamstring pulls. One clinical observation indicated that hamstring pulls are more common with short, stocky people who may innately have tight hamstrings. Proper stretching, warm-ups and caution will help prevent any sudden force that might pull the hamstring area unnecessarily. Please remember that not all people can stand up, bend over with their knees straight and put their palms on the ground. For some of us it is impossible and that's o.k. as long as you stretch out slowly to your maximum and the muscles are warm before working out.

Be aware that bouncing during warm-ups is not good. Gentle, consistent stretching is the best. Remember, too, that if people are learning or warming up for the splits, this should be done very slowly, especially if they are young. The piphyseal plates of the ischial tuberosities are not calcified until about the 18th year and there is the possibility of avulsing (breaking off) a portion of the lower pelvis. All of this is to say that you must be carefully when stretching the hamstring and quadriceps area. Use good common sense as these muscle groups are extremely large and strong and once injured, can take a great deal of time to heal properly.

> *"More and more these days I am seeing cheerleaders wearing knee braces. They not only seem to inhibit their skill execution but the braces are almost an ugly distraction from their spirited faces. What types of activities predispose cheerleaders to knee problems and how can they be prevented?"*

KNEES

Cheerleaders are predisposed to knee injuries just like any other athlete is. Neither hockey, gymnastics, football, soccer, basketball, baseball or cheerleading are necessarily good for knees. Generally speaking, any type of activity where there is a locking and a rotating of the knee will predispose you to a knee injury. The knee is most stable in a close packed or a locked position. At this point the leg is straight, the muscles and ligaments tight and the femur flush with cartilage between it and the tibia. If you take this particular knee, apply a medial to lateral force or an anterior to posterior force, something has to give way. Generally this is a ligament or tendon at the knee joint. Cheerleaders who are bases for pyramids or partner stunts usually have locked knees. Partner stunts in which bases rotate their foot for stability can cause this type of problem. A person coming out of a stunt to the ground can "land wrong" and have a problem. You can no doubt think of dozens of other possible situations that could cause a knee problem. They are too numerous to mention here, but being aware to avoid situations where the knee is locked and then required to rotate should help. With respect to cheerleaders wearing "ugly" knee braces, if there is a significant injury that needs to be protected or supported, then a brace is effective. If not, there is nothing that takes the place of hard work and exercise to strengthen the knee joint and the surrounding musculature.

> *"It seems like every year, just as basketball season gets underway and my skills are really getting good, I get sidelined with a terrible case of 'shin splints. How can I help from losing out on two to three weeks of cheering each year?"*

SHIN SPLINTS

"Shin splints" is another catch-all term commonly used to describe pain in the lower leg. It is necessary to get a specific diagnosis so the appropriate treatment can be started. Some common examples of lower leg problems are posterior medial pain, tibial pain, anterior tibial compartment pain, lateral compartment pain, fibular pain, posterior compartment pain and popliteal artery entrapment. Let's assume, for discussion's sake, that the injury you have a question about is posterior medial pain, the most common type of pain experienced by cheerleaders. The pain runs inside the length of the tibia, the large bone in the lower leg, and towards the back of that area in question. Many things can cause this type of pain but probably since you alluded to this occurring at the start of the basketball season, the change in surface is the culprit. Coming from the soft field or the cinder track to a relatively hard gym floor or even cement will increase the stress on the lower leg musculature and cause irritation. This problem can be helped by making sure that your shoes have adequate arch support with good shock absorption. The old "cute cheerleading shoe" with the thin sole is highly outdated and can cause lots of problems. If your shoes are okay, then you may want to consider strengthening your tibialis anterior muscle, the large muscle on the front of your lower leg. Some experts feel that an imbalance between that muscles group and your cal musculature can be the problem. Sometimes tape and anti-inflammatory drugs will help, as well as resting the muscles as much as possible (i.e., not jumping or tumbling for a while). Should you still have pain that limits your performance, you need to see a physician and make sure there is no damage to the bone itself, such as a stress fracture. "Shin splints" can be very painful, but with proper treatment, they can be managed so that you don't lose two to three weeks of cheering each year.

> *"I always have one or two cheerleaders on my squad who have 'weak ankles' and seem to have a sprain at the most inopportune times, such as the day before competition or a big game. Are there any exercises which can help strengthen ankles?"*

ANKLE SPRAINS

Ankle sprains, as we talked about earlier, can be very painful and hard to avoid. Strengthening is the best way, along with being very careful, to prevent ankle sprains. The problem is that there are no major muscle bellies that run across the ankle joints, there are only ligaments and tendons of the muscles. However, these muscles should be strengthened to help stabilize the tendons and in turn stabilize the ankle. Heel raises, toe raises, resisted inversion and eversion all help to accomplish this. An excellent ankle strengthening program can be found in the reference book mentioned above on sports medicine. Remember that shoes with good medial and lateral stability at the heel will help greatly because they will balance the foot when landing from a jump, stunt or tumbling pass.

> *"Every year at camp we experience problems with the heat. What can we do to acclimate or prepare ourselves at home? Also, what can we do at camp to help combat heat-related injury?"*

HEAT RELATED INJURY

In speaking about heat related injury, it is important to know some physiology facts. As the athlete exercises, the body temperature obviously rises in a warm environment. The bigger the athlete, or the more subcutaneous fat present, the more heat is produced. The body tends to throw heat off in three ways: through cooling of the skin; through sweating, which is the most important mechanism; through the lungs, and also conduction, convection or radiation. It is important to remember that heat cannot easily be evaporated from the skin in an area of high humidity. It is also important to know that the body is actually being heated by the environment with temperatures above 99 degrees F and also if water loss from sweat and perspiration is not replaced, then dehydration can occur. These principles are extremely important in heat related injuries. It is important that when you prepare for camp, you must acclimate yourself to some degree. One way to do this is to begin with short workouts in the heated environment in which you will be competing. As time progresses, increase the length of time that you work out in this heated environment, always being careful to replace any fluid that is lost at short intervals and if any signs of dizziness or headaches or nausea occur that the practice should be stopped. Some general rules for fluid replacement, which tends to be the single most important item in preventing heat injury, is to have a great deal of water on hand. Small amounts of electrolyte substances as in sugar, in any form, may delay absorption in the tissue and is not necessarily good for athletes exercising less than two hours. One suggested fluid intake plan might be for two hours before practice the athlete should drink approximately one liter or 34 ounces of water. Fifteen minutes before practice the athletes should drink approximately 13 to 17 ounces of water and then every 15 to 30 minutes during practice there should be at least 13-17 ounces of water consumed. Again, after practice 5 to 6 large glasses of water or fluid should be taken to prevent any dehydration. The water should be cool water, not necessarily cold and certainly not warm. Such problems as heat exhaustion and heat stroke were discussed in the definitions. It is important to remember that fluid replacement and acclimation are the two major things that should be addressed when working in conditions of severe heat. As far as problems at camp, if a regime of acclimation and fluid replacement is established throughout all the workouts the camp should not be any more difficult to handle than the daily practices.

> *"Foot injuries tend to be problematic with regards to cheerleading, pom-poms or dance. Can you describe some of the more common ones and their treatment?"*

FOOT INJURIES

Three fairly common foot problems are plantar fasciitis, Morton's neuroma and metatarsalgia. The first, plantar fasciitis, is an inflammation of the fascia on the plantar or bottom aspect of the foot. Generally this is caused by chronic irritation of excessive pronation which results in microtears of the fascia itself. People with high arches or markedly tight plantar fascia are susceptible to this type of injury. It commonly presents with pain and tenderness in the arch of the foot and with pain that radiates forward from the arch and sometimes the heel particularly with the first steps early in the morning. Treatment normally consists of ice massage in combination with anti-inflammatory medications. It is important that excessive pronation be corrected either with taping or orthosis. Rarely is surgery necessary and injections of cortical steroids should be used prudently.

The second problem mentioned, Morton's neuroma, is a term that describes a small neuroma which generally presents toward the head of the metatarsals in the foot. It is commonly caused by a shearing force secondary to a hyper-mobile foot that tends to have excessive pronation during the propulsive phase of late-mid support and early take of either with walking, jumping or running. Generally it

presents itself acutely with an electric type shock pain radiating from the fore foot down to the toes usually in the third and fourth toes but it can occur between any two. The athlete rapidly removes the shoe from the foot to obtain relief, generally taking the pressure off this will help. In its chronic stage it presents as a dull discomfort under the foot and on palpation is localized to the metatarsal interspace or the spaces in between the metatarsal heads. The treatment for this particular problem can be helped initially with a metatarsal bar which is used to relieve the pressure on the heads of the metatarsals as well on the nerve and some kind of in-shoe orthotic to prevent excessive pronation as prescribed by an orthotist. If these do not produce satisfactory results, local anesthetic, perhaps cortico-steroid injection, can be used around the neuroma itself. Generally surgical excision is a last choice, but it may be necessary in some resistant cases.

The third problem or metatarsalgia is defined as a pain across the metatarsal heads. Generally this can include a large number of problems, such as calluses, blisters, corns and even sesamoditis which is generally seen as the tissues surrounding the sesamoid bones are inflamed just below the great toe. Metatarsalgia generally presents with tenderness and sometimes swelling in a localized area over the head of the metatarsals on the plantar aspect of the foot. Upon passive dorsiflexion of the

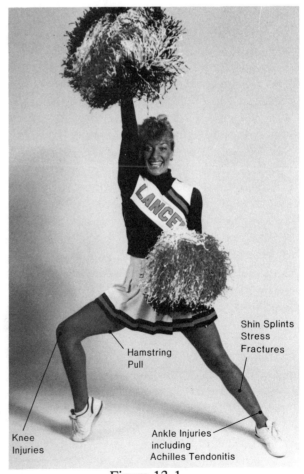

Figure 13-1

161

foot and palpation over the head of the metatarsals there is significant discomfort. Treatment initially is ice and anti-inflammatory medication and generally non weight bearing. Sometimes the posterior splint of some kind with gentle toe extension and walking on the heel can be used. As the athlete returns to either performance or competition, it might be noted that the toe should be taped in plantar flexion to avoid any excess dorsi flexion or stretching of the tendons over the metatarsal joints. It's also noted that sometimes a small felt padding underneath the head of the metatarsals might help alleviate some of the pain. Generally the best treatment for this is non weight bearing and rest. The athlete should participate in activities that will not stress this particular area, such as swimming and cycling and allow the area to heal either with the anti-inflammatory medication or non weight bearing.

WHY CONDITION?

Regular conditioning is one of the best things you can do for yourself . . . for general fitness and for developing good cheerleading skills. Exercise strengthens your heart. It burns calories like there is no tomorrow. But before you break a sweat, let's get one thing straight.

Good cheerleading skills are not something you buy. And you're not going to find a magical pathway. Fitness is work. Hard work. A commitment to improve yourself. Much, much more than just looking good.

Conditioning is about "being good." It's about believing in yourself and what you can become. Getting out there and doing what it takes to reach your peak.

So the next time you start to exercise, hit it a little harder than before. Don't settle for anything less than your best. Believe in your potential. Improve yourself, impress yourself. Reach your peak performance!

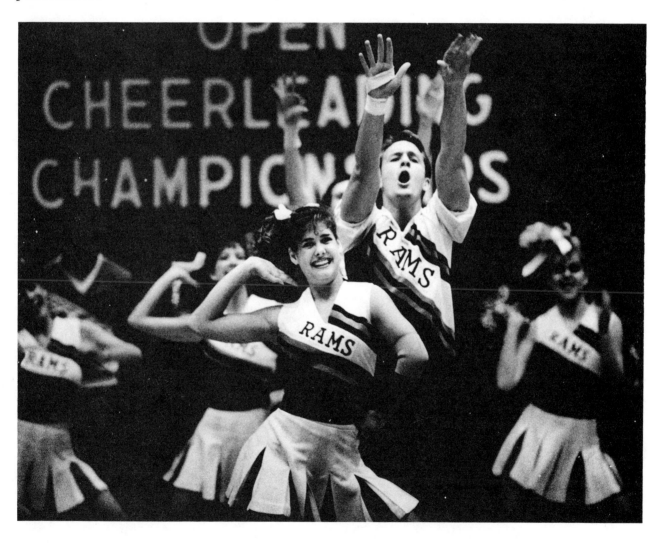

Contributors

Christy Lane
* National free lance dance choreographer
* Certified International Dance Exercise Association and American Coaching Effectiveness Program
* Author, *All That Jazz, The Complete Book of Jazz Dance*
* Trained in Los Angeles and New York City
* Former cheerleader and ICF camp instructor
* Former member, Palm Springs Dance Company
* Artistic Director, Jazz Dancers, L.T.D. and Class Acts Dance Academy
* Member National Dance Association and American Alliance of Physical Education, Health and Dance
* Guest speaker at Universities 38 States

Debra Knapp
* B.A. Education and Physical Education
* Cheerleading coach and camp instructor
* Coordinator, Indiana Coaches Conference
* Aerobic dance trainer, Aerobics Dance Company (California)
* Choreographer, Indiana Power Lifting Championships
* Member, International Dance Education Association
* Former cheerleader and ICF camp instructor
* ICF National Staff Training Director

Denise Gator
* B.S. Physical Education
* M.S. Exercise and Sports Sciences
* Certified Strength and Conditioning Specialist
* University of Arizona Strength and Conditioning Assistant Coach, 14 sports including cheerleading, gymnastics, varsity men's basketball
* Co-Chairperson Women's Committee, National Strength and Conditioning Association
* Competitive Diver, Pan American Gold Medalist, AIAW National Champions, American Cup Champion and former NBC Commentator

Scott Cusimano
* M.S. Physical Therapy, Sports Medicine and Exercise Physiology
* B.S. Psychology, Pre-Physical Therapy
* Head coach and program director, Olympiad Gymnastics Club, St. Louis, Missouri
* Former head coach, Kippers Gymnastic Club, Oklahoma
* Director, ICF Physical Skills and Conditioning Programs
* Former Southeastern Louisiana University varsity cheerleader and ICF camp instructor
* ICF National Staff Training Director

Keith Englekey
* B.S. Physical Education
* B.S. Exercise and Sports Science
* Director, University of Arizona Adult Fitness Program
* Former United States Olympic Committee Consultant

Jeff Newman
* B.S. Physical Therapy
* B.S. Biology
* Clinical Assistant Professor at University of Texas, Southwestern Medical Center
* Licensed Physical Therapist, Texas, Colorado
* Private practice Physical Therapy and Sports Rehab Clinic, Fort Worth, Texas
* Cheerleading injury prevention and rehab consultant
* Member of American Physical Therapy Association
* Member, Private Practice Section, A.P.T.A.
* Member, Orthopedic and Sports Section of A.P.T.A.